Latina and Hair Care

Shine and Health: Your Essential Guide to Gorgeous Hair

Catalina Charpentier B.

ISBN: 978-1-961176-15-7 (eBook)

ISBN: 978-1-961176-16-4 (Pbk)

ISBN: 978-1-961176-17-1 (Hardback)

Publisher: ARTEMIX BEAUTY, Owasso, Oklahoma Website: www.artemixbeauty.com

Instagram: @artemixbeauty Facebook: @artemixbeauty

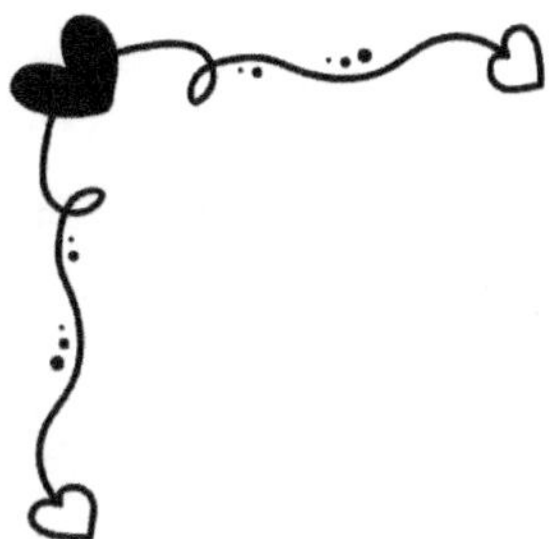

JUST FOR YOU

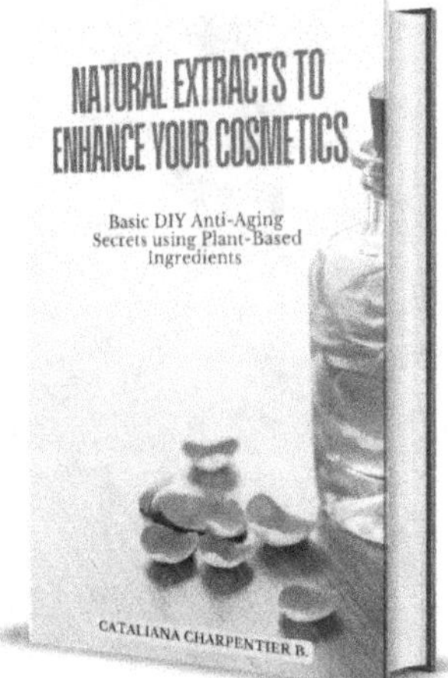

A FREE GIVEAWAY

Learn about Natural Anti-Aging Extracts

www.artemixbeauty.com

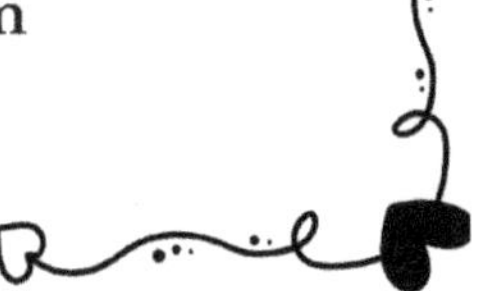

Contents

Introduction

Frizz, knots, tangles, and split ends are some of the never-ending battles we have with our hair. Hair care is an essential part of daily grooming, but for Latinas, the significance of hair is deeply rooted in culture and identity. Latina hair is diverse, ranging from thick and curly to fine and straight, and requires specialized care to maintain its health and beauty. With so many products and conflicting information available, it can be difficult to know where to start! If you've ever wondered:

- What type of hair do I have?

- What are the best products for my hair?

- How can I improve my hair's health?

Then there's good news. It is possible for your hair woes to end. Embracing healthy hair practices and your hair's natural texture is key to making every day your best hair day. Your hair's natural texture is already beautiful, and this book offers a comprehensive guide to Latina hair care to help you bring out the best in your hair.

Latina hair can be classified as straight, wavy, curly, or coily; more details on this are provided in chapter one. It is often overlooked that each hair type requires specific attention and care to maintain its health and beauty. We can't treat curly hair the same as straight hair. It simply won't work. That's because curly hair tends to be dry and frizzy and requires regular deep conditioning treatments and hair oils to keep it moisturized. Straight hair can become greasy and flat, requiring light hair products and frequent washing to look its best. A different haircare approach is needed for different hair types, so figuring out your hair type is an important first step to achieving runway-ready hair.

When we know our hair type, it is simply a matter of choosing the right products and styling techniques for our hair. Hair care couldn't be simpler. It is recommended to use hair care products designed specifically for Latina hair. These products are formulated to provide additional nutrition and moisture to the hair and help maintain its natural texture and shine. Knowing how to choose hair care products based on hair type and texture is a game changer. Don't worry; this book will help you with that if you're not sure where to begin. A good place to start is with healthy hair practices.

Healthy hair practices, such as regular washing, conditioning, and trimming, are extremely important to maintain the good health of your hair. It's a good idea to develop a consistent hair care routine and stick to it. Take the time to learn what your hair likes and avoid using excessive heat or chemicals on the hair whenever possible. Heat and chemicals can cause damage and lead to breakage. Instead, try to use natural hair masks and oils to nourish and strengthen the hair. Your hair will thank you!

Hair is not just a physical attribute. So why not embrace your hair's natural texture and celebrate the uniqueness of Latina hair culture? In addition to the practical advice and tips on hair care, you'll find step-by-step instructions on creating different hairstyles. Whether you are a Latina who has struggled with her hair care routine or someone who is interested in learning more about hair care, there's something for you on these pages. Without further ado, let's get started on the journey to healthier, beautiful hair!

One
Hair Types in the Latin Community

Latina hair is as diverse and beautiful as Latinas themselves. From sleek and sexy to lusciously coily (and everything in between), there is no denying that hair is a woman's crowning glory. Whether you prefer getting your hair done by that one tia who does everyone's hair or you prefer to dedicate a day to going to the salon, hair days are events in their own right. We could spend hours on end taking care of our tresses, laughing, and listening to all the juicy neighborhood gossip. What's not to love about that?

Hair means a lot to Latinas; I'd dare say more so than most other communities, as Hispanics account for 16% of all the sales in the hair care category in the U.S. market (Roeschley, 2015). We love our hair, and rightly so! It is the hallmark of femininity, but did you know that hair was also used as a symbol of resistance throughout history? One famous example comes from West Africa. During the years when the Transatlantic slave trade was in full swing, slaves would adopt cornrows as a clandestine communication method, intricately weaving maps and escape plans into their beautiful locks (Khalfe, 2022).

As revolutionary as hair can be, many Latina women might still hear the dreaded phrase *pelo malo,* or "bad hair." Latinas are under great pressure to look presentable at all times, which means "bad" hair has no place in our lives. As a result, we spend many hours fixing our supposedly unruly hair, chasing the coveted *pelo lacio* norm (Castañon, 2017). It doesn't help that the media does not do enough to represent the LatinX community. Of the 100 top-grossing films in 2016, only a scant three percent had Hispanics in leading roles (Smith et al., 2017). The whitewashing of LatinX characters leaves much to be desired, so we spend inconceivable amounts on blowouts and hair care products to achieve "good" hair. Thankfully, the narrative is changing, and Latinas are learning to embrace and celebrate their beautiful, natural hair!

Pelo malo is losing its meaning, becoming a made-up term that is used to suppress something beautiful. And it's about time! Your hair, whether it is curly, wavy, straight, coily, or something in between, is magnificent. Different hair types have different needs, and proper hair care is important for maintaining healthy and beautiful hair. Of course, knowing our hair type makes the process a lot easier!

Getting to Know Different Hair Types

Hair types are classified based on the shape and size of the hair strand. The shape of the follicle and the angle at which the hair grows out of the scalp will determine how curly our hair will be. Hormones and medications can influence our curl pattern to some extent, but the blueprint for our follicle shape is locked in our DNA, which reasserts itself every time our hair goes through its growth cycle (Stanborough, 2019-b). This means each hair type will have unique characteristics, requiring specific care and styling techniques to remain healthy, manageable, and beautiful.

Hair types are generally divided into four categories (straight, wavy, curly, and coily), which can be subdivided into subcategories based on the tightness of curls. Classifying hair types can be a complex business, and it is entirely possible for an individual to have natural hair with a mix of characteristics. With that being said, let's take a closer look at the hair types and the characteristics that define them.

Straight Hair

Sometimes referred to as Type One hair, this is hair with no natural curl. The strands may vary in thickness and texture, but they will fall from root to tip without a single wave, just like Demi Lovato's hair. This hair type has a tendency to look flat and can become oily easily, so it is best to avoid adding hair care products with oil in them. It's not recommended to add heavy butters or serums to your hair care routine, as they can make straight hair oily very quickly. Texture sprays and dry shampoos are the straight-haired woman's best friend, as they help to add body and reduce the appearance of oil on the strands. Layered haircuts also help to add extra movement and give the illusion of a fuller head of hair. Straight hair is the most common hair type among people of European descent. It is generally easy to manage and style, requiring minimal effort. Popular hairstyles for straight hair include sleek ponytails, bobs, and blunt cuts.

Wavy Hair

Wavy hair is characterized by hair strands that form an "S" shape. Wavy hair falls between straight and curly hair, with some strands being straighter while others have more defined waves. This hair type is common among people of mixed ethnicities and is often associated with a carefree, beachy look. Popular hairstyles for wavy hair include loose waves, textured bobs, and beachy waves. Hydration is the secret to keeping wavy hair bouncy. To bring the best out of this hair type, we need to look for hydrating hair care products. This hair type can easily be divided into three subcategories based on the curl pattern.

Type 2A

A gentle, tousled texture can be seen, but the hair appears fairly straight from the roots to your mids (eye level). From the mids downwards, a loose and undefined wave can be seen, just like Gisele Bündchen's hair. The hair tends to be fine, and it is really easy to straighten or curl. In order to preserve the natural wave, it is recommended to avoid oil-based and creamy products. An airy mousse or light gel will help to preserve the texture, which is so easily lost.

Type 2B

Picture those gorgeous, beachy waves that Jenifer Lopez has, and you'll have a good idea of what this hair type looks like! Type 2B hair has a more defined S-shape than 2A and will need a little more effort to straighten. This hair type is absolutely stunning with the balayage trend, and you'll normally only need a spritz of salt spray to create that airy, beachy look. The battle of the frizz is real, so moisturizing products and frizz-fighting gel is the wavy girl's best friend.

Type 2C

This hair type is easy to spot! The consistent tight waves look like they've been made with a curling wand and start close to the crown. Shakira has this hair type. Just like Type 2B, this hair type is prone to frizz when the weather is damp. This hair type tends to be thick and dry, so moisturizing products such as deep conditioners and leave-in cream serums are recommended. Anti-humidity products can help to keep the dreaded frizz away, locking the gorgeous waves in place.

Curly Hair

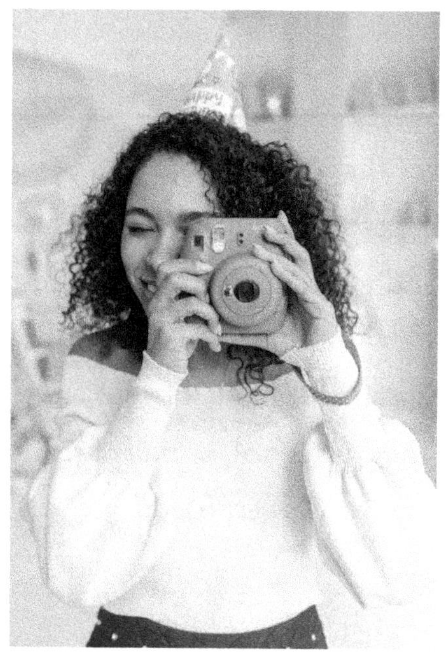

This hair type has a tendency to become dry and prone to frizz, making it a bit of a challenge to maintain. Curly hair is common among people of African and Mediterranean descent. Popular hairstyles for curly hair include afros, twists, and defined curls. Moisturizing products are necessary to keep this hair type healthy, and any detangling is best done when the hair is still wet. If you're looking for a fresh haircut, make sure to go for something that won't texturize the ends, as this will give curly hair a very frizzy appearance. Just like wavy hair, this hair type can be classified into three subcategories.

Type 3A

Soft, S-shaped curls form loose loops, just like Salma Hayek's hair. Brushing usually wrecks the curl definition, leaving us with a very frizzy, floofy appearance. Girls with this hair type should steer clear from wearing their hair in a ponytail or bun for prolonged periods, as this ruins the curl definition and can lead to thinning at the hairline. Contrary to popular belief, this hair type is not coarse and is fairly easy to style in its natural state. It's advised to steer clear of heavy butters and oils, as these will weigh the curls down. Gels and creams that offer moisture and curl definition will help to keep these soft curls enticingly bouncy.

Type 3B

This is a mix of big curls and stretched-out spirals, like Mariah Carey's hair. The curl circumference tends to be the size of a Sharpie marker, but you might have looser curls at your crown and tighter curls in the nape of your neck. Frizz control and moisture is a priority here, so whipped mouses are a good option. It's also recommended to use a microfiber towel and satin pillowcase to minimize frizz. Silicones and sulfates are the enemy of curly hair and can contribute to dry, damaged hair.

Type 3C

Lupita Nyong'o's tight, springy hair is the perfect example of this hair type. These corkscrew curls easily coil around a drinking straw but are prone to frizz and breakage. The hair tends to be fine, dry, and fragile, so we'll need butters and leave-in conditioners, which will provide moisture throughout the day. It is best to air dry these delicate strands.

Coils

This hair type is very delicate and needs to be handled with extra love and care. Coily hair is characterized by hair strands that form tight coils or corkscrews and is often referred to as "kinky" hair. Coily hair is the most fragile and prone to damage, as it tends to be dry and prone to breakage. Popular hairstyles for coily hair include afros, twist-outs, and Bantu knots. Preserving moisture and strength is the top priority for ladies with this hair type. As with wavy and curly hair, coily hair can be classified into three distinct types.

Type 4A

Tight, small curls that become super long when stretched are typical of this hair type. Yaya DaCosta's hair is the perfect example here. The strands are fine and will need a lot of moisture. Deep conditioning butters, masques, and creams are your best bet to preserve this hair type's natural beauty. It is also recommended to wear the hair in loose, wash-and-go styles and to steer clear from protective styles as these may prevent us from moisturizing the hair properly.

Type 4B

The curl pattern does something very interesting here! Instead of forming an S-shape like the types mentioned before, Type 4B forms a Z-shape. The result is a hair texture that is less defined, with a soft and thick cotton-like feel. Leave-in oils and creams are your best option to protect the integrity of these delicate strands. One way we can add some definition to the hair is to accentuate the natural curl pattern with shingling. This technique requires detangled wet hair and liberal amounts of leave-in conditioner. The hair is then sectioned into four parts. Using your fingers, gently work curl cream or gel down the length of each curl, gently twisting the strands around the index finger.

Type 4C

This hair type has loads of volume of curl but no desirable curl pattern. That's because the curls are tightly clumped together, just like Esperanza Spalding's hair. This hair type does not become oily easily, but it is super fragile. Frequent nourishment in the form of rich conditioners is important to keep this hair type healthy.

Understanding Porosity and Density

We'll often hear hair professionals talk about the porosity and density of hair. When they are talking about hair density, they are referring to the number of hairs we have on our heads. If you can see your scalp without parting your hair, it's likely that you have low-density hair. There are a number of things that can influence the number of hairs we have on our heads, including stress, nutrition, menopause, and hormones during pregnancy (Stanborough, 2019-b). It's always a good idea to keep an eye on the products we are using and if they are impacting hair density. If we have low-density hair, it's best to use light mousses for volume and texture sprays, as heavy products can flatten the hair. High-density hair can benefit from butters and creams for improved shine and manageability.

When hair professionals refer to the porosity of hair, they are talking about cuticles. Every strand of hair is made of three layers, with the cuticle being the outermost layer (Yang et al., 2014). Much like overlapping roof tiles, this layer of dead, scaly cells helps to keep the fragile inner layers of the hair intact. How smooth, frizzy, or shiny our hair is will also tell us how healthy the cuticles are! When our hair is damaged, these overlapping layers become jagged and open up. Just like a roof with missing roof tiles, these damaged layers allow more moisture to enter the hair shaft. There are three different hair priorities that can result from this:

- **Low porosity**: Hair tends to take a long time to dry, and product buildup is a common occurrence. Low porosity hair has a habit of being less responsive to chemical and heat treatments and is commonly seen in individuals with chemically straightened hair and those with naturally curly and coily hair. Low-porosity hair needs long-lasting moisture, so look for hair masks with moisturizing ingredients like jojoba ester oil to help keep the cuticle hydrated.

- **Medium porosity**: Hair that is classified as medium porosity absorbs moisture and products fairly well, and chemical treatments have predictable results. This is the ideal hair porosity and indicates healthy cuticles.

- **High porosity**: This hair has a tendency to become frizzy, breaks easily, and feels dry. This is typical of hair that has been exposed to chemicals or physical stress. While this porosity type responds well to hair dye, it is unable to retain moisture for long. With this porosity type, it is important to moisturize and protect the strands from breakage and frizz. Lightweight, moisturizing ingredients like argan oil can help to add luster and smoothness to locks.

Got a few minutes and a bowl of water? That's all you'll need to check your hair porosity. Simply lay a few strands of your hair in a bowl of water. Check on the hair a few minutes later. What do you notice? If your hair is floating, then it's low porosity. High-porosity hair will sink as it can absorb more water. Healthy cuticles are the secret behind gorgeous hair! This means our hair care routine should focus on minimizing damage and keeping hair moisturized.

Cutting down on chemicals and the use of heat tools will help, but we need to pay attention to the hair's moisture balance. This is where knowing your hair porosity can help a lot! Product buildup can easily weigh down low-porosity hair. A hair care routine making use of lighter products to create volume, such as milks and mousses, and a clarifying shampoo can inject new vitality into low-porosity hair.

Why pH Matters

When it comes to maintaining the health and strength of hair, pH can make a drastic difference in how hair looks and feels. The natural pH level of hair is slightly acidic, hovering between 4.5 and 5.5 on the pH scale (What is Hair pH and Why is it Important For Your Hair, 2022). Coloring, bleaching, shampoos, and treatments can push our hair's natural pH balance towards the alkaline.

Damage occurs when the pH of the hair is forced toward the alkaline end of the spectrum. When this happens, the cuticle begins to open up, impacting the hair's strength and health in the long run, resulting in problems like breakage and frizz. Not to mention that a more alkaline environment may possibly lead to dandruff.

So the secret to healthy hair is maintaining an optimal pH level. Shampoos and conditioners that are pH balanced help maintain that delicate pH balance for shiny, strong locks. Look for shampoos that are formulated with citric acid. This acidic formula serves to strengthen weakened bonds in the hair, leaving our tresses smoother and less prone to frizz.

Hair care is important for maintaining healthy and beautiful hair. Proper hair care involves regular washing, conditioning, and styling. Good hair care practices can prevent damage and breakage, promote hair growth, and maintain hair health. That's because we preserve the health of our cuticles. Each hair type requires specific hair care practices, such as the use of specific products and tools.

Neglecting hair care can lead to hair loss, dryness, breakage, and other hair problems. Hair neglect can happen in many ways. By using the wrong product for your hair type, and improper washing, styling, and brushing techniques, the cuticle becomes damaged. By investing a little bit of time and effort in our hair care, we can prevent many hair dilemmas in the first place! Proper hair care ensures that our hair looks and feels its best. I'll spill all the secrets of choosing the best hair care products for your hair type in the next chapter!

How to Choose the Best Latina Hair Care Products

Imagine the sun kissing your skin as the wind playfully flirts with your dress. You feel as glamorous as the movie stars you adore, but will your hair hold up? When our hair becomes a tangled mess, it is usually a sign that we are using products that don't cater to our hair's needs. Some shampoos might leave the scalp feeling itchy and dry, while other products can leave our hair hanging in limp clumps. It's a hair-raising situation that can steal the thunder from our glamorous moments, but it can be prevented with a little bit of knowledge.

Before selecting a shampoo or conditioner, we need to understand what the product does and how it relates to our hair and scalp type. In the previous chapter, we spoke about hair types. You have most likely already identified your hair type. Now you can build on that knowledge by getting to know your scalp.

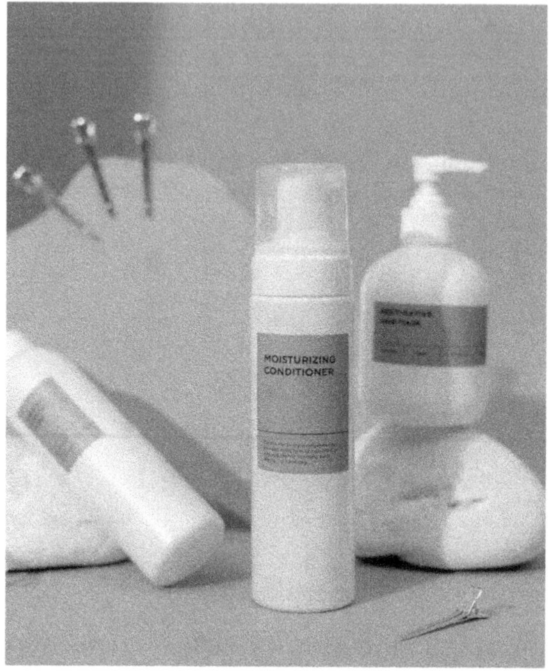

Whether your hair sticks straight or falls into wispy ringlets, your shampoo should be chosen based on scalp health. The skin on the body and scalp are the same, so if you have dry skin on your legs and arms, chances are that your scalp will be dry too. The shampoo you choose should be suitable for your skin type; otherwise, it can lead to an itchy and uncomfortable scalp. To prevent the hair from becoming weak and brittle, we need to use a pH-balanced shampoo. Preserving the pH on the scalp and hair can help prevent cuticle damage, helping our hair grow longer and stronger. Other considerations we need to keep in mind when selecting shampoos and conditioners include thickness, oiliness, and color treatment.

- **Thickness of hair:** People with thin hair (the scalp can easily be seen) will benefit from using shampoos that contain more cleansing agents. Flat hair can be challenging, so volumizing shampoos can help to fluff up those fine tresses. People with thick hair will need to use a shampoo that contains equal amounts of cleansing and moisturizing ingredients. That's because thick hair tends to be drier and can gather dirt quicker.

- **Oiliness of hair:** If you've got dry hair, your best bet is to use a shampoo rich in nourishing ingredients like coconut oil, grape seed oil, argan, or avocado oil to keep those locks lush and soft. Those with oily hair won't need to use any special shampoo, but they need to be on the lookout for dandruff. An oily scalp is a veritable feast for yeast (which produces flakes), so the best treatment is an anti-dandruff shampoo.

- **Color-treated hair:** Color-treated and chemically processed hair needs extra gentle care. Ideally, we want to use a shampoo that will cleanse the scalp but won't strip away or fade hair color. Look for shampoos containing antioxidants (such as vitamin E or green tea) to protect and nourish these fragile tresses.

It may take some trial and error to find the product that works for your hair, but the rule of thumb is this: Choose your shampoos for the scalp and your conditioners for the length of your hair (Importance of Choosing the Right Shampoo for Your Hair Type, n.d.). So if your scalp is oily, but you have dry ends, it is best to use a shampoo that can address the oily scalp while you hydrate the dry ends with a suitable conditioner.

Natural Latina Hair Products

Many Latina hair products are made with natural ingredients, such as oils, herbal extracts, and other organic ingredients. These products are usually gentle on Latina hair and provide essential nutrients to keep hair shiny. Natural hair products typically do not contain silicones, but it can take a bit longer for the results to show. In recent years, there's been a growing trend among Latina women to embrace natural products, especially personal care items. Data from NielsenIQ indicates that nearly a quarter (21%) of Latina women are willing to embrace more natural products (Manso, 2021). That's great news for our hair (and the environment, to some extent). Natural hair care products are filled with ingredients that are kind to the hair follicle and gentle on the scalp.

If you are diving head-first into the sea of natural hair care products, know that the results can take a few weeks to a few months to show (Cook, 2019). Natural products can be pricier than their mass-produced counterparts, but we can see this as an investment in ourselves. We are worth every penny if the end result makes us feel good! Consistent care and some patience are needed, but the end result will be lively, shiny locks that every hairdresser instinctively wants to style! Various oils and extracts are used in natural products, including:

Olive Oil

Dry, brittle, and frizzy hair giving you those 80s vibes? Then olive oil may be the magic ingredient your hair care routine is lacking. The oil from this small, tasty fruit is filled with fatty acids, vitamins, minerals, and antioxidants, making it the perfect choice to smooth hair fibers, lock in moisture, and restore shine (The Ancient Powers and Benefits of Olive Oil for Hair, n.d.). When applied to the scalp, olive oil can help to clear dandruff and treat itchiness.

Olive oil hair masks tend to work well on coarse, dry, chemically processed, or damaged hair (Raypole, 2019). If you have fine hair or an oily scalp, it is best to use this mask very sparingly. To make a basic DIY olive oil mask, you'll need the following:

- Extra virgin olive oil. How much you'll need will depend on your hair. Some people need as little as two tablespoons of oil, while others may need a quarter cup. If you want to treat the ends of your hair only, you may need as little as one tablespoon.

- Gently warm the oil and stir in any essential oils (such as rosemary or peppermint) that you are using. Massage the oil into the scalp and hair while it is warm. An applicator bottle can make this process easier. Section your hair. That way, it is easier to apply the mask.

- Cover the hair with a shower cap after the application is finished and allow it to sit for at least 15 minutes. If it's your first time using an olive oil mask, you may want to consider washing it out after 15 minutes. Olive oil can leave hair greasy sometimes. If it does not leave your hair greasy, feel free to leave the mask on for 30 minutes next time.

- Shampoo and complete your hair care routine as per usual.

For dry, damaged hair, an olive oil mask twice a week may be beneficial. If the oil turns your hair oily, consider using it sparingly. For those with acne-prone skin, it is advised to wash the skin after the hair mask has been applied.

Coconut Oil

The right balance of protein is vital to keep hair strong and healthy. By stretching one of our strands and observing it closely, we can determine if the hair needs more protein or moisture. If the strand stretches more than usual and feels stiff and dry, it's likely you'll need to introduce moisture into the hair follicles. If the strands stretch without breaking you'll need more protein. Hair may also feel limp. This is where coconut oil can be very beneficial, as it is one of the best oils around to reduce protein loss in our hair (West, 2021). Whether your hair is chemically processed or one hundred percent natural, coconut oil's unique chemical structure allows it to be easily absorbed into the hair, protecting it from additional damage. This versatile ingredient is typically used as a mask, conditioner, or scalp treatment to encourage shiny, luscious hair. Here's how you can harness coconut oil's powers to revitalize dull hair.

- Combine coconut oil (two tablespoons to a quarter cup, depending on the amount and length of hair) and one tablespoon of apple cider vinegar. Add two tablespoons of honey and a few drops of your favorite essential oil.

- Coat hair evenly with the mixture and allow it to work its magic for 15 to 20 minutes. Rinse, shampoo, and complete your hair care routine like normal. This treatment can be used once a week to restore shine and softness to hair.

Almond Oil

Thinning hair stressing you out? Then almond oil might be the hair rescue you need! This oil is rich in vitamin E, has excellent emollient properties, and can be used on all hair types to nourish hair and promote new growth (Catcher, 2021). The results? Soft, manageable hair that is less likely to break.

Argan Oil

A powerhouse of an ingredient, this oil is filled with antioxidants and fatty acids (mainly oleic and linoleic acid) to lubricate and protect hair follicles (Santos-Longhurst, 2019). Products containing argan oil can help to reduce frizziness, styling damage, and sun damage, impart a healthy shine, and prevent dryness. Moreover, argan oil is good for the skin and can help prevent skin problems that can lead to hair loss, such as psoriasis and seborrheic dermatitis (scaly patches of skin accompanied by dandruff). The result? Less breakage and shedding for a head full of sleek, bouncy hair.

Argan oil is an excellent choice for hair care. One of the best ways to utilize this beautiful oil is by creating a hair serum. A serum is a concentrated product that helps retain moisture. Argan oil is an ideal base ingredient for a serum or leave-in conditioner due to its lightweight texture and natural botanical properties. You can experiment with your own preferred carrier oils and essential oils to make a personalized treatment for your body; just make sure to use a maximum of two percent dilution of essential oils (Hannah, 2018). To make the serum, you'll need:

- 2 oz organic argan oil

- 12 drops of organic lavender essential oil

- 6 drops of organic rosemary essential oil

- 6 drops of organic basil essential oil

Carefully pour argan oil into a 2 oz cobalt blue glass dropper bottle. A funnel can make things easy. Add the essential oils and tightly screw the top on the dropper bottle. Shake well to combine. This serum is now ready to use. Remember to shake the serum before every use to ensure the oils are combined.

To use the argan oil serum, towel dry your hair after washing it and apply a pea-sized amount of the serum to the ends of your damp hair. Rub the serum briefly between your hands to warm it up and ensure you're not using too much. Use it daily for a glossy, vibrant look.

Green Tea

Hair loss and increased shedding are challenges that many of us will have to cope with. Fortunately, there is an easily available ingredient that can help turn bad hair days into a distant memory. Green tea is the secret to preventing severe hair loss, and its anti-inflammatory nature leaves the scalp feeling clean. It also has the added benefit of combating bacteria and fungi on the scalp that may lead to hair fall. Most significantly, green tea contains catechins (antioxidants) which can help reduce DHT (dihydrotestosterone), preventing hair loss (Gupta, 2020). Experience the benefits of green tea with this easy rinse.

- Brew some green tea for 15 minutes and allow the brew to cool down. The idea is to have enough tea to give your hair and scalp a proper rinse. Pour the cooled mixture into a spray bottle or applicator bottle for ease of use later.

- After shampooing, apply the cooled green tea to the scalp. Massage the scalp for a few minutes and rinse out. This rinse can be repeated up to three times a week.

Peppermint

Not only does this ingredient smell wonderful and leave the scalp with a fresh, tingly feeling, but it can also prevent our scalps from becoming dry and itchy (White, 2018). The menthol present in peppermint is a vasodilator, meaning it can help improve blood flow to the scalp. Improved blood flow means better-nourished hair and less hair fall.

Best of all, peppermint oil promotes hair growth (Oh et al., 2014). That's great news if you've been looking for ways to give your hair a bit of a boost. Peppermint oil can benefit all hair types when used correctly and safely. Direct application should be avoided as it can cause irritation, and those with essential oil allergies or sensitive skin or scalp should either avoid it or do a patch test before use.

Peppermint oil is particularly helpful for oily hair as it clarifies and cleans without stripping away natural oils. It also balances sebum production, leaving hair nourished and hydrated without feeling heavy (Gould, 2022). Many hair care products, including shampoos, conditioners, and scalp treatments, contain peppermint oil as an ingredient.

There are several ways to use peppermint oil for hair care, such as massaging it into the scalp or diluting it with a carrier oil like jojoba or argan oil. One can also mix it with shampoo or make a DIY hair mask with coconut oil to stimulate blood flow. Peppermint essential oil is easily obtained from natural food stores or online. Always dilute this essential oil, as it may cause irritation if used in too high concentrations. To hydrate a dry scalp, consider using coconut, almond oil, apricot kernel, or grapeseed oil as the carrier oil.

To use the essential oil, dilute two to three drops in a tablespoon of carrier oil. Vigorously massage the mixture into the scalp for two to three minutes, starting from the front of the scalp and rubbing in circular motions.

Periodically dip the fingers into the essential oil mixture while massaging the sides of the scalp, the back of the hair, and the middle of the scalp. This application may enhance blood flow to the scalp (Nall, 2018). Allow the oil mixture to sit for up to 10 minutes before washing and styling as normal. Repeat the application once a week to encourage healthy hair growth in the long run.

Rosemary

Touted by hair gurus as the ultimate hair growth secret, this ingredient is the hair follicle's best friend. Researchers compared rosemary's hair-growing powers with those of minoxidil (a medication that is used to treat hair loss), and the results were nothing short of jaw-dropping. Over a six-month period, the researchers found that rosemary performed just as well as minoxidil in increasing hair count (Panahi et al., 2015). Rosemary owes its awesome hair powers to its anti-inflammatory and antioxidant properties (Bradshaw, 2022). Just like peppermint, this ingredient promotes circulation, allowing oxygen and nutrients to reach the hair.

Want to add rosemary essential oil to your hair care routine? Here are a few easy ways to do it:

- **Make a mask:** Mix five drops of rosemary essential oil with a teaspoon of carrier oil, such as jojoba or coconut oil, and massage evenly into the scalp. Leave the oil on for at least 10 minutes before shampooing and completing the haircare routine.

- **Mix it with hair products:** Add about five drops per ounce of product, such as shampoo or conditioner, and use as usual. Alternatively, add three drops directly to a dollop of product before use.

- **Make a DIY shampoo:** Follow a recipe to create shampoo and add essential oils, including rosemary, for their health and beauty benefits. Dilute the oil with a carrier oil or other product to avoid skin irritation.

Before using rosemary essential oil, avoid contact with the eyes and dilute it with a carrier oil or other product to prevent skin irritation. The safety of using rosemary essential oil during pregnancy or while breastfeeding is unknown, so caution is advised (White, 2022).

There is no shortage of natural ingredients to address all our hair problems; however, the ones mentioned here are widely used and generally easy to get a hold of. By selecting natural hair care products with ingredients that our hair loves, we'll be one step closer to growing and maintaining show-stopping hair.

Chemicals for Latina Hair

We use chemical products on our hair every day. Whether these chemicals come in the form of shampoos and conditioners or dyes and straighteners, there's an abundance of chemicals used in hair care products to keep our manes healthy and shiny. These chemicals aren't all bad and can be very useful if used properly. On the flip side, low-quality products and the overuse of chemicals can lead to dry, damaged hair. Some chemicals should be avoided from the start, though. The list of chemicals to avoid in the table below should help you considerably on your healthy hair journey.

Products Specially Formulated for Latina Hair

There's no denying that hair care is one of the driving forces behind Latin American beauty. The category is constantly evolving. Some products are specifically formulated for Latina hair. These products usually contain natural ingredients and specific chemicals to help keep hair healthy and shiny. These products are usually more expensive than non-specially formulated Latina hair products but generally provide better results. If we investigate this market segment a bit deeper, we'll find that there's a bit more to Latina hair care products than meets the eye.

According to research, some 43% of Brazilian women are looking for products that can fix damaged hair (Pitman, 2018). Knowing how meticulous Latinas are when it comes to personal care, it is unlikely that the blame falls solely on the overuse of hot tools. The high demand for damage repair products is due to a combination of harsh environmental factors (pollution, UV exposure, water quality, and so on) and various styling trends.

It is not unusual for Latin hair products to address a variety of hair and scalp conditions, with some treatments designed to be used at night. Hair care is as serious as skin care, and by using the right product for the right purpose, Latinas can make a big difference to their hair.

The Importance of Choosing Products Specific to Your Hair Type

Choosing hair care products that are specifically designed for your hair type is essential to achieving and maintaining healthy, beautiful hair. Hair type refers to the natural texture and thickness of your hair, and different hair types have unique characteristics that require specific care. We discussed the different hair types and their characteristics in the previous chapter. If you have curly hair, you need a product that can define and enhance your curls without weighing them down. Similarly, if you have fine hair, you need a product that adds volume and thickness without leaving your hair greasy or weighed down. Finding the products that your hair likes can feel like an uphill struggle, but it's a struggle that pays dividends in the long run.

When we use products that are not suited for our hair type, a range of issues can result. Dryness, dullness, and breakage are common consequences, but other issues can arise too. For example, using products designed for straight hair on curly hair can lead to our curls losing their definition and becoming frizzy. If we use products that are too heavy on fine hair, the hair will be weighed down and look greasy. So by selecting our hair care products to correspond to our hair type, we are one step closer to banishing bad hair days for good!

Ingredients to Look for in Latina Hair Care Products

When choosing hair care products, it's important to pay attention to the ingredients. Certain ingredients can help nourish and strengthen your hair, while others can cause damage or irritation. Here are some ingredients to look for in Latina hair care products:

- **Argan oil:** Argan oil is a natural oil that helps to moisturize and nourish hair. It is a useful ingredient for dry or damaged hair. The oil helps to reduce breakage, split ends, and everyday damage, making it an ingredient that promotes fuller, thicker hair. The antioxidant activity in argan oil may help to provide protection against UV damage from ultraviolet rays (Santos-Longhurst, 2019).

- **Shea butter:** Shea butter is a natural moisturizer that helps to soften and strengthen hair. This ingredient works well for coily and curly hair. The secret to shea butter's moisturizing powers lies in its high concentration of fatty acids and vitamins. These fatty acids include linoleic, oleic, palmitic, and stearic acids, making shea butter a great choice for smooth, glossy hair fibers (Watson, 2019). Interested in using shea butter on your scalp? Section off tiny bits of hair. This makes it easier to massage the shea butter in. Use circular motions to distribute the product. If your hair is very dry or damaged, consider applying shea butter to the lengths of your hair and using it as a treatment before shampooing (How to Use Shea Butter for Hair and Skin, n.d.).

- **Coconut oil:** Coconut oil is a natural oil that is great for all hair types. The ingredient helps to moisturize and protect hair and has other benefits. Coconut oil can restore luster to dry hair, tame frizz, and is filled with fatty acids to aid in hair health (Wong, 2022). This versatile ingredient can be found in many hair care products, including conditioners, masks, treatments, and styling gels.

- **Aloe vera:** This natural ingredient is deeply moisturizing. It's great for dry or damaged hair and can help to combat hair fall. That's because aloe vera is rich in vitamins A, E, and C—important vitamins contributing to healthy cell growth. Folic acid and vitamin B12 are also present in aloe vera gel. Both of these nutrients play an important role in preventing hair from falling out (Watson, 2023).

- **Jojoba oil:** Jojoba oil is technically not an oil. It is a wax ester that has a similar composition to the natural oils that our skin secretes, making it a good call for all hair types! The oil is filled with oodles of antioxidants and vitamins, and when applied to hair, it leaves it feeling softer and looking shinier (Brady, 2019). Jojoba oil can be easily included in your hair care routine. Use it as a hot oil treatment and allow it to work its magic for 20 minutes or more. You'll need one tablespoon of oil for short hair and two tablespoons for longer hair (White, 2017). Distribute the oil evenly from root to tip and shampoo, condition, and style as normal afterward.

Types of Shampoo, Conditioner, and Styling Products

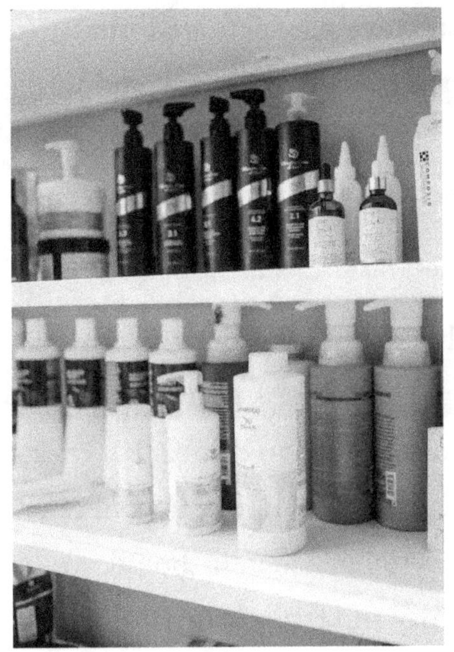

Most of us use shampoo and conditioner on autopilot, giving little thought to how they might impact our hair's health. As it turns out, an intentional hair cleansing ritual is a vital part of having healthy, voluptuous hair. No fancy gadgets or expensive bathroom upgrades are needed. Taking care of your hair starts by selecting the shampoo, conditioner, and styling products that are designed for your hair type. After that, we should tailor our hair-washing routine to suit our needs. Let's take a closer look at the different kinds of shampoos, conditioners, and styling products available.

Shampoo

Shampoo is a hair care product that helps to cleanse hair and remove dirt and oil. Shampoos are designed with different purposes in mind, and your scalp is one of the most important things to consider when selecting a shampoo. If some shampoos left your mane an untamable, frizzy mess, then perhaps it's time to take a closer look at the label. Here's a breakdown of what to expect from shampoos we'll find in a typical store:

- **Anti-breakage shampoo:** These products are formulated for hair that has been over-processed, damaged, and weakened. The cleansing ingredients are gentle and restore the pH balance of the scalp and hair, leaving hair healthier and stronger.

- **Clarifying shampoo:** This shampoo is designed to strip away product buildup on the hair. Think of this product as a scalp and hair detox and can be used to combat the effects of pollution, oil, and product buildup, restoring vibrancy to our locks. Just like any detox product, it should not be overused, as it can lead to a dry and frizzy mane.

- **Moisturizing shampoo:** A lack of moisture is one of the biggest reasons why many people have weak, dry hair. The oils that our scalp produces are necessary to lock moisture in, but sometimes it needs a helping hand. Moisturizing shampoos help to restore moisture to the hair follicles and impart a healthy, shiny look. It's a lifesaver if you have dry and brittle hair! If you have an oily scalp, then it is recommended to steer clear of this product, as it will create a bigger oil problem on your head.

- **Purifying shampoo:** This is not the same as a clarifying shampoo. Where the clarifying shampoo focuses on the removal of product buildup, purifying shampoos help combat hair woes by fighting dandruff. The product usually has cleansing, shooting, and antimicrobial benefits, making it an excellent choice to keep our shoulders free from those pesky flakes.

- **Regular shampoo:** Just plain old shampoo that is designed to clean the scalp of oils and dirt. This type of shampoo is ideal if you don't have any special hair needs.

Generally speaking, if you have dry hair and scalp, it is best to stay away from volumizing and fortifying shampoos, especially shampoos that list sulfate on the ingredient list. If you have an oily scalp, then clarifying shampoos can help, but it should not be overused. For hair and scalp that is neither oily nor dry, it is best to select a product based on your hair type and the desired results.

Conditioner

Conditioner is a hair care product that helps to moisturize and detangle hair. Whether we are styling our hair or simply throwing it into a messy bun, daily wear and tear can result in hair damage. A shampoo alone does not cut it. Shampoos are designed to clean the scalp but do not replenish lost moisture. That's the conditioner's job. When used with every wash, conditioner can help keep hair moisturized, reduce frizz, and improve the manageability and general condition of hair. This is why we shouldn't skip the conditioner, even when we are in a hurry. Not all conditioners are the same or should be used the same way. These products include:

- **Conditioner:** Just regular old conditioner that is meant to stabilize the pH of the scalp after shampooing. This product helps to add moisture and shine to hair and assists in detangling.

- **Deep conditioner:** Can be used instead of a conditioner after shampooing. It helps to stabilize the scalp's pH but has the added benefit of enhancing moisture retention. If hair is dry or chemically damaged, deep conditioner or conditioning masks can help to restore life to your locks.

- **Leave-in conditioner:** This lightweight conditioning formula is used after the hair is shampooed and conditioned to manage frizz, detangle hair, and manage moisture. Leave-in conditioners are especially useful to refresh textured and curly hair.

- **Co-wash conditioner:** These are cleansing conditioning products that replace shampoo and conditioner on some wash days. It is a product that is meant to be rinsed out fully, as it contains a small amount of cleansing agent. Co-washes are deeply hydrating, making them ideal for dry, damaged, chemically processed, curly, or coily hair.

Styling Products

Styling products are used to help shape and hold your hair in place. Most styling products will not damage our hair when applied as intended (Gavazzoni Dias, 2015). When using styling products, we do run the risk of drying our hair out; there's no escaping that. Some styling products might dissolve the natural oils on the hair, while others could leave a residue. There are different types of styling products, including mousse, gel, and hairspray.

Mousse

Mousse is particularly great for those with curly hair, as it can help define curls without leaving them looking stiff or crunchy. When applied correctly, mousse can give curls a bouncy, defined look that lasts all day. It can also be used to tame frizz and add shine, making it a versatile styling product for a range of hair types (What is Hair Mousse and How to Use It, n.d.). To use mousse, start with damp hair and apply a golf-ball-sized amount of product to your hands. Work the product through your hair, starting at the roots and working your way out to the ends. For best results, use a diffuser attachment on your hair dryer to help enhance curls and add volume.

Overall, mousse is a great choice for those looking to add volume, shine, and definition to their hair. It is a versatile product that can be used to create a wide range of hairstyles, from sleek and sophisticated to playful and curly.

Gel

Hair gel is a versatile tool that can be used to create movement and hold hairstyles in place. Styling gels come in different formulations and can add texture, shine, and body to the hair. A medium-hold gel is perfect for creating a playful bedhead look, while stronger hold gels are great for achieving a sleek, slicked-back style.

Gels are available in varying levels of hold, ranging from light to extra-strong. Light-hold gels are great for adding subtle texture and definition to the hair, while medium-hold gels are perfect for creating more defined styles that still have some movement. Strong and extra-strong hold gels are ideal for keeping hair in place all day long, making them a popular choice for formal events or elaborate updos.

While gels are great for short hair, they may not be the best option for longer hair. This is because gel can make longer hair look stiff and crunchy, which can be unflattering. However, if you have longer hair and still want to use gel, opt for a lighter formulation and apply it sparingly to avoid a stiff, unnatural look.

Overall, hair gel is a versatile styling product that can help you achieve a wide variety of looks. Whether you're going for a playful, tousled style or a sleek, sophisticated look, there's a gel out there that's perfect for your needs.

Hairspray

Hairspray formulations protect hair against heat and humidity, and we all know how humidity can mess with a cute hairstyle! The product is formulated to work on the majority of hair types. It can hold all sorts of complex hairstyles, tame unruly curls, and eradicate frizz for a beautifully put-together hairstyle. Different hair sprays have different purposes, so we need to take note of that for optimal results.

- **Regular hairspray**: This type of hairspray is designed for basic styling and to keep flyaways in check. It typically has a medium hold, making it perfect for everyday use.

- **Texturizing hairspray:** This hairspray adds volume and texture to the hair, making it ideal for creating beachy waves or tousled, messy styles. It's great for all hair types and is particularly useful for fine or limp hair that needs a bit of a boost.

- **Finishing hairspray:** Finishing hairspray is the last product used in hairstyling and is designed to hold your hair in place. It typically has a strong hold, making it perfect for more complex hairstyles that need to stay put. However, it can also make hair stiff and crunchy, so it should be used sparingly.

- **Volumizing hairspray:** As the name suggests, this hairspray is designed to add volume to the hair. It typically has a lightweight formula that won't weigh the hair down, making it perfect for those with fine or limp hair.

- **Freeze hold hairspray:** This type of hairspray is similar to finishing hairspray but has an even stronger hold. It's perfect for locking a hairstyle in place, and it's often used by stylists responsible for runway looks or elaborate updos.

- **Shaping hairspray:** Shaping hairspray is designed to help hold a hairstyle in place while also improving the hair's texture and manageability. It's often used in conjunction with other styling products to achieve the desired look.

- **Thermal hairspray:** Thermal hairspray is designed to protect hair from heat damage caused by hot styling tools like curling irons and straighteners. It typically contains ingredients like keratin and silk proteins that help strengthen and protect the hair while also holding the style in place.

There are many different hairsprays, and choosing the right one for the job can take hairstyles from flat and uninstructed to runway-ready. Similarly, choosing the right shampoo, conditioner, and other styling products can make a big difference in the health of our hair.

Choosing the right shampoo, conditioner, and styling products for your hair type can make a big difference in the health and appearance of your hair. By understanding your hair type and choosing products with the right ingredients, you can achieve beautiful, healthy hair. Of course, thermal hair spray can only go so far in protecting our hair from heat treatments. Whether it's the hot tools or the hairdryers, heat damage is a battle we are all too familiar with. In the next chapter, we'll get to know our nemesis well.

Three

The Dangers of Excessive Heat Treatments for Latina Hair

Temperature can drastically alter the appearance of our hair. Whether we live in a cold, dry climate or are addicted to the curling iron, the effect of temperature on our hair is clear to see. Some hair growth myths would have us believe that temperature can influence hair growth. This is not true. Temperature extremes can make it challenging to retain the full length of our hair, but there is not enough evidence to support the idea that they can impact growth rates. For most people, hair growth happens at roughly half an inch per month, but this does not mean that the temperature is off the hook. There are other ways it can mess with a perfect hair day.

Too much heat turns hair brittle, leaving us with the joys of split ends. A common source of excessive heat exposure is the use of curling irons, hair dryers, and flat irons. While these tools are safe when used properly, they can have a negative impact on hair over time. Some hot tools don't allow us to adjust the temperature, seriously damaging the hair on a molecular level. The keratin in hair undergoes a change at temperatures over 300°F. At these temperatures, α-keratin converts into β-keratin, resulting in weak hair that's lost elasticity (How Does Heat Damage Hair? n.d.). Considering that a flat iron can reach temperatures of 250°F to 425°F, it is not surprising that heat tools are the leading cause of damaged hair. There's more sad news on top of this because there's no going back for the keratin that underwent the change, meaning the damage from heat can become a permanent fixture if we're not careful. Heat can be useful when used correctly. Some treatments need heat to open the cuticle scales, making them more effective.

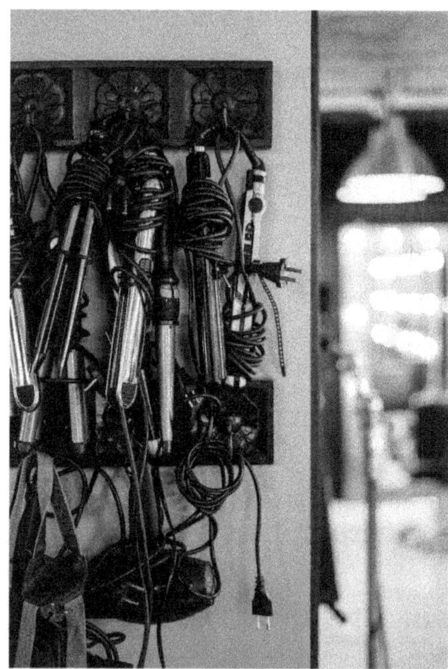

Excessive heat treatments for Latina hair can be very dangerous. This is because Latina hair is drier and more fragile than typical hair, making it more vulnerable to damage caused by excessive heat. The long-term permanent damage that can be suffered includes hair burns, loss of shine and elasticity, and decreased hair length and thickness. These damages can be disastrous for hair health, and the results can be difficult to reverse. In order to avoid these negative effects, it is essential to remember a few things when using heat on Latina hair.

- Always use a heat shield before starting the treatment, and choose a suitable temperature for your hair.

- Avoid drying your hair too much with hot air, and avoid overuse of irons and curling irons.

By following these simple steps, you can minimize the dangers that excessive heat treatments hold for Latina hair.

Signs of Heat Damage

Over the years, the use of hot tools to style hair has become an essential part of daily life, and it is easy to see why. Whether it is bouncy curls or a sleek, elegant look, thermal hair styling can give us quite the confidence boost and spice up our look for any occasion. Unfortunately, heat can do more than lock curls in place; it can cause serious damage to hair, especially if we use low-quality tools, use high settings, or ignore recommended practices to prevent damage. Heat damage can leave several visible signs on your hair. Here are some common signs of heat damage to look out for:

- **Split ends:** When your hair becomes dry and brittle due to excessive heat, it can cause the ends to split. This is one of the most common signs of heat-damaged hair. Split ends indicate that hair has become weak and lost its elasticity. That's because the disulfide cysteine bonds (which make up the proteins in our hair) break down with heat, weakening the hair. Using low-quality hot tools without a thermal heat protectant is usually the leading cause of split ends, but other factors can contribute to the problem.

- **Breakage:** Heat damage weakens hair, making it more prone to breakage. You may notice broken strands of hair or excessive shedding. If you notice excessive hair loss when brushing or detangling, it could be a sign of heat damage. Keep in mind that shedding is a natural part of the hair growth cycle and that we normally shed between 50 and 100 hairs daily (American Academy of Dermatology Association, n.d.-c). Hair strands continuously collect damage until they are shed, so frequent exposure to high temperatures is not a good idea if we want to keep our locks shiny and bouncy. Excessive hair loss can also be a sign of a stressful event or illness recovery, so it should not be ignored.

- **Dryness:** Excessive heat can strip your hair of its natural oils, leaving it dry, dull, and prone to frizz. Frequently exposing your locks to high temperatures causes the hair to lose moisture and can crack the cuticle layer. Roughly 15% of our hair's composition is water, so evaporation caused by high heat makes hair more vulnerable to damage (7 Signs of Heat-Damaged Hair & 3 Ways to Revive It, 2023).

- **Changes in texture:** Heat damage can alter your hair's natural texture, making it appear flat, lifeless, or limp. Since hair loses elasticity when it becomes heat damaged, your tresses are more likely to feel uneven and frayed at the tips.

- **Lack of elasticity:** Heat damage can reduce the elasticity of your hair, making it more difficult to style and manage.

- **Frizziness:** When hair does not align with surrounding hair strands, it creates an irregular, frizzy texture. Heat damage is one of the main causes of a frizzy mane, but it is not the only one. Genetics, humidity, and heat styling wet hair all contribute to a frizzy appearance.

It's not possible to reverse hair damage because the protein bonds have been permanently altered. Prevention is much better than cure in this case, but there are ways we can repair damaged tresses without going for a big haircut. If you simply can't give up your curling wand or flat iron, then consider investing in good-quality heat tools with adjustable heat settings. This allows for better temperature control, giving us the cute hairstyles we desire with minimal heat. Another step you can take is to use a thermal heat protectant before using hot tools and to avoid using that flat iron or curling wand on hair that's not fully dry. Split ends should be trimmed every two to three months as well. It's advisable to adjust your hair care routine to ensure that you're using gentle and nourishing products on your hair. On days that you do decide to use thermal styling tools, follow these steps to minimize damage:

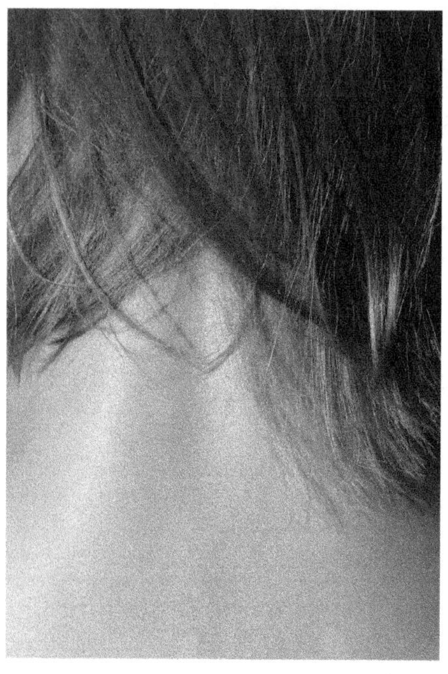

Step One: Cleanse

The ingredients in your shampoo matter, as we discovered in the previous chapter. So using a shampoo that is suited for your hair type will help eliminate some hair troubles. Sulfate-free shampoos are a fantastic option, especially when we are embracing our natural hair. Even though every head of luscious hair is different, it is possible to overuse (or underuse) shampoo. If the scalp feels itchy, gets greasy fast, or if your hair is exceptionally frizzy, then it's high time to scrutinize those ingredients on the label and adjust your hair-washing routine.

Step Two: Deep Treatment

If you plan to use heat tools, it's best to use a moisturizing and reconstructive treatment beforehand. The treatment helps soften hair and smooth frizzy, textured hair. Applying the treatment for 30 minutes to an hour should do the trick, depending on your hair's porosity. A mask or deep treatment that contains shea will give curly hair the maximum amount of moisture it needs before heat styling.

Step Three: Protecting

Using a heat protector is beneficial for a few reasons. The product helps to keep the style in place longer and acts as a barrier between the heat tool and the hair fiber. Apart from smoothing the cuticles, heat protectants can help prevent hot spots in the hair. These "hot spots" are areas of concentrated heat, which can weaken the hair. Argan oil is an effective ingredient to protect naturally coily and curly hair from the ravages of heat, so make sure to check the label of your favorite heat-protectant product.

How Heat Affects Hair Texture, Porosity, and Strength

Excessive heat can alter the texture and porosity of your hair, leading to further damage. The cuticle coats the outer layer of every hair strand, much like the shingles on a roof. These shingles overlap in healthy hair, giving it a smooth appearance and feel. When we apply heat to hair, the cuticle opens up, making the hair more porous and allowing moisture to escape. Healthy strands can withstand temperatures of up to 232°C (449 °F) on occasion (Heat-Damaged Hair; How Heat Can Affect the Health of Your Hair, n.d.), but when we crave a blowout, playful curls, or a super-sleek look frequently, the damage becomes inevitable.

Underneath the cuticle, we'll find the cortex. In this layer of the hair strand, we'll find keratin, which gives hair its shape. Keratin forms bonds that help lock in moisture and provide strength to the hair shaft. One of the bonds is a hydrogen bond—a bond that is notoriously easy to break with heat. This can cause hair to lose its natural curl or wave pattern, giving it a straighter and flatter appearance. Extended heat exposure can dry the cortex, leaving us with fragile, brittle hair. One way we can reduce the effects of heat on hair is to use our thermal styling tools on their lowest heat settings to reduce the risk of heat damage. Heat tools can help us create many playful and cute hairstyles, but they can seriously fry our tresses if we're not careful.

The Impact of Heat on Hair Growth and Health

If you thought the evils of hot tools stopped at giving you a few split ends, you're in for an unpleasant surprise. Excessive heat can also have a negative impact on your hair's growth and overall health. When our hair is exposed to excessive heat, we run the risk of damaging the hair follicles, which can slow down hair growth and lead to hair loss. If you've noticed that your hair is thinning, it might be a good idea to take better care of your follicles.

Have you ever inspected some of your shed hair and noticed a little bulb on the one end? That's the base of the root that anchors the hair into the scalp. While the follicle is alive, it constantly produces cells that will eventually die and become our hair. Even though the strands are dead, the root is very much alive and needs to stay healthy. When hair is exposed to excessive heat, it can damage these follicles, which can slow down hair growth or trigger hair loss. Follicles are easily damaged when we use heat tools close to the scalp. Furthermore, heat damage can cause inflammation and damage to the scalp, which can impede hair growth and cause discomfort. Over time, excessive heat can weaken the hair and cause long-term damage that may be difficult to reverse.

Fortunately, making some simple changes to your brushing and styling routine can help preserve the integrity of your hair. The frequency of hair washing, whether we brush our hair while it is wet, the towel, and the styling products we use all have an impact on hair and follicle health. Additionally, try to cut down on the use of heat tools and hold your hairdryer a distance of 15 centimeters (six inches) or more from the hair (BosleyMD, n.d.). Allowing the hair to air dry naturally can help improve follicle health and reduce the resulting hair loss we experience as well.

It's essential to be mindful of the amount of heat you apply to your hair and take steps to protect it from heat damage. By recognizing the signs of heat damage and understanding how heat affects your hair's texture, porosity, strength, and growth, you can take steps to minimize the damage and keep your hair healthy and beautiful. In the next chapter, we'll take a look at how you can level up your hair care game by embracing natural hair care techniques.

Four
Natural Latina Hair Care Techniques

We spend much of our adult lives on the noble quest to uncover the secret to shiny, silky hair. Many natural hair care techniques are suitable for use on Latina hair. Who knows? Perhaps the secret to taming those stubborn flyaways has been hiding in your pantry all along. Maybe your abuela or tia shared their hair care secrets with you as you were growing up. Whether they encouraged the use of oils to moisturize hair, oil-based treatments to nourish and strengthen hair, the use of herbal extracts to revitalize, or the use of homemade masks to moisturize and restore hair, there's no doubt that they were onto something. Oils are one of the best treatments for Latina hair. Coconut oil, olive oil, and castor oil are great options for moisturizing hair. These oils can be applied directly to the hair or mixed with other ingredients, such as honey, to create a nourishing mask.

Oils aren't the only champion in haircare. Herbal extracts are also an excellent choice for Latina hair care. Herbs such as mint, sage, thyme, and rosemary have properties that help strengthen and revitalize hair. These herbs can be mixed with water to create a nourishing hair lotion.

Homemade masks are another open secret in the LatinX community. These are a great way to nourish and restore hair. They can be created by mixing natural ingredients such as honey, yogurt, eggs, and essential oils. These masks are applied to the hair and left on for a few minutes before rinsing with warm water. In this chapter, we'll explore effective hair care techniques that are definitely abuela-approved!

Gentle Cleansing Techniques

Cleaning the hair is an essential part of any hair care routine. It involves removing dirt, excess oil, and product buildup from the hair and scalp. Most people would reach for any shampoo to do the trick, but that does not give our tresses the love and care they deserve. Here are some natural and gentle cleansing techniques that can be used to enhance the natural beauty of Latina hair.

- **Co-washing:** Co-washing, short for conditioner washing, is a technique where a conditioner is used to cleanse the hair instead of shampoo. This technique is particularly useful for those with dry, curly hair that tends to be frizzy. Gentle hair care couldn't be easier as this technique requires a single product. As the conditioner used contains a small amount of cleansing agent, it is important to rinse the product out properly. To co-wash, wet the hair thoroughly and apply a generous amount of conditioner to the hair. Use your fingertips to give yourself a scalp massage as you work the product into your hair and scalp. Allow the conditioner to sit on your hair for a few minutes before rinsing thoroughly. Co-washing is useful to prevent dry, brittle hair as it retains our natural oils while getting rid of dirt. It can also help reduce frizz, improve hair texture, and make the hair easier to manage.

- **Apple cider vinegar rinse:** An Apple Cider Vinegar (ACV) rinse is a technique used to cleanse the hair and scalp while balancing the pH levels. ACV is a natural astringent that helps remove product buildup and excess oil from the hair. There are many benefits to using ACV, ranging from improved shine and scalp health to stronger hair (White, 2023). Hailed as a panacea for many health problems, it's not surprising that ACV has found a home in the haircare market.

To do an ACV rinse, mix one part apple cider vinegar with two parts water in a spray bottle. After shampooing, spray the mixture onto the hair and scalp. Using your fingertips, massage the ACV into the hair and scalp and let it sit for a few minutes. Rinse thoroughly with warm water. ACV rinses can help restore the hair's natural pH levels, which can make the hair appear smoother, shinier, and more manageable. Why does pH matter? Because dull, frizzy, or brittle hair tends to be more alkaline, which impacts the hair's overall strength and integrity. By using a natural product like ACV, we can restore the pH levels on our scalp and hair to improve hair health. It can also help soothe an itchy, flaky scalp and promote hair growth, so ACV (when properly diluted) is definitely one of those abuela-approved remedies!

Conditioning Technique

The second step to hair washing is conditioning the hair. Unless we are co-washing, it is not recommended to skip this step. Shampoos and ACV cleanse the hair from sweat, dead skin cells, and product residue, but the conditioning step leaves hair feeling soft and manageable. It also prevents damage to the hair shaft by locking in moisture. Regular, run-of-the-mill conditioners are formulated with fatty alcohols, humectants, and oils to impart softness and shine to hair.

Not only is dry, unconditioned hair a pain to style but it can be filled with static! Unless we have a young cousin who we can entertain with static and a balloon, it's safe to say that we don't want our hair rising to the ceiling. Conditioner helps by clinging to the hair and making it less staticky. That's only a regular conditioner, though. For Latinas whose tresses need an extra boost, deep conditioning might be the answer.

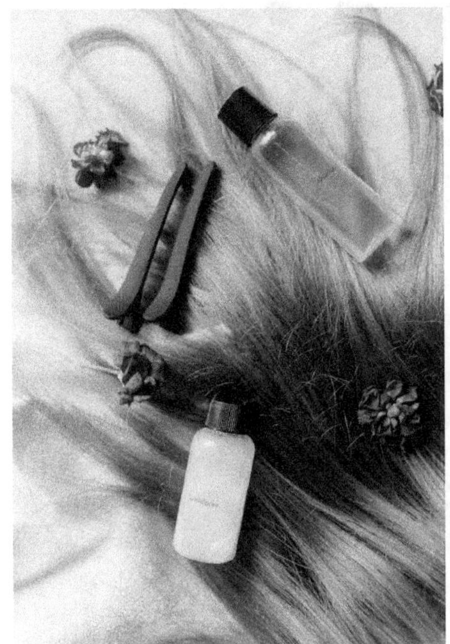

Deep conditioning is a technique where a thick, nourishing conditioner is applied to the hair and left on for an extended period. The conditioner you use should complement your hair type. This technique is particularly useful for those with dry, damaged, or chemically treated hair, as it will impart oodles of moisture to parched strands.

To deep condition the hair, start by washing it with a clarifying shampoo to remove any buildup. Use a generous amount of product and focus your application on the mids and ends of the hair. This section of hair is the oldest and tends to be more damaged, so it will need extra gentle care. Cover the hair with a plastic cap or towel and let the conditioner sit for at least 30 minutes or overnight. Rinse thoroughly with warm water to remove the product.

Deep conditioning can help nourish and strengthen the hair, making it less prone to breakage and split ends. It can also improve hair elasticity, enhance hair texture, and restore moisture to the hair.

Hot Oil Treatment

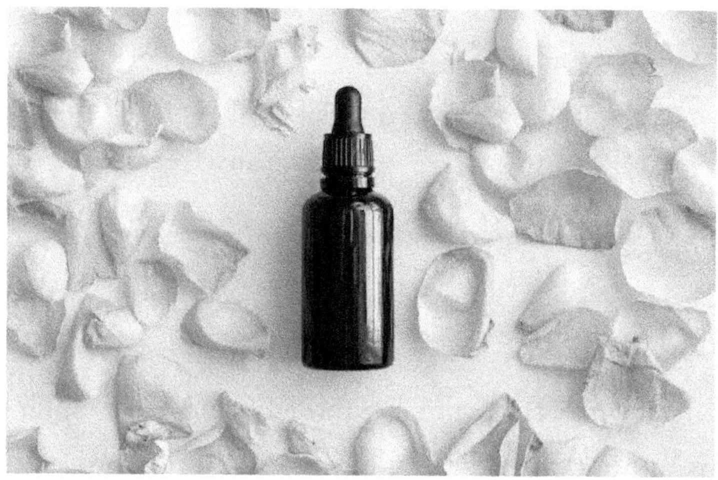

A hot oil treatment is a technique where warm oil is applied to the hair to penetrate the shaft and provide deep conditioning. It's a stylist-recommended method of restoring life to hair and is very simple to do. But before we take a look at how to do the treatment safely and effectively, we'll answer some frequently asked questions about hot oil treatments.

How Does Hot Oil Help Your Hair?

Warm oil seals the cuticle by giving the hair follicle extra moisture. This can help prevent and, in some cases, repair split ends. Additionally, hot oil can help solve dry scalp issues by deeply moisturizing the skin. The foundations of a proper hot oil treatment are quite easy to remember. It only needs a scalp massage and time! So if you want to strengthen your hair and restore luster from root to tip, go ahead and spoil yourself with your favorite hot oil. Your hair will thank you.

Do Hot Oil Treatments Cure Dandruff?

Let's get one thing straight: a flaky scalp and dandruff are not the same thing. This is an important distinction because they are treated differently. Dandruff is usually linked to an overproduction of skin cells (Dry Scalp vs. Dandruff, n.d.), whereas a flaky scalp is the result of dry skin. Remember all those times your abuela or tia scolded you to moisturize your ashy skin? That's pretty much what is happening on the scalp. Just like ashy skin, the scalp becomes dry due to a lack of natural oils. This leaves the scalp feeling tight, uncomfortable, itchy, and stinging. The result is usually frizzy and dull-looking hair, which is understandable, as not enough moisturizing oils are produced to lubricate everything. That's where hot oil treatments can become a lifesaver! By deeply moisturizing the scalp, hot oil can help to eliminate a tight, itchy, and flaky scalp for flake-free shoulders.

Will Hot Oil Treatments Be Beneficial for Curly, Textured, and Frizzy Hair?

Absolutely! Curly, coily, and textured hair types may benefit the most from a hot oil treatment, as these hair types tend to be more porous. To use hot oil treatment effectively on thin hair, one must apply a smaller amount to the scalp, as the oil can be overpowering. Hot oil treatments can be especially beneficial during the dry winter months, as they can deeply condition the hair. Hot oil treatments can help to soften and protect textured hair, leaving it shiny and easy to manage.

What Precautions Should I Take With Hot Oil Treatments?

There are a few things we need to keep in mind before drenching our locks in oil. First, the temperature of the oil should not be too hot; otherwise, you'd scald the scalp. Also, hot oil treatments should not be applied to dirty hair. We want the cuticle to be open to encourage maximum absorption of the oil, so the best time to apply hot oils is when the hair is wet. After the oil has worked its magic for at least 30 minutes, it can be shampooed out. When using oil on your scalp for the first time, it is encouraged to do a patch test first. Pick a spot close to the scalp to observe the skin's reaction (if any) easily. This patch test will reveal if the oil is safe to use. If there are no adverse reactions, feel free to use the oil.

How Do I Know If Hot Oil Is The Right Thing For My Hair?

That's an easy one to answer! Anyone who has normal, dry, or frizzy hair can benefit from hot oil treatments. The only time hot oil treatments are not advised is when you have a damaged scalp or thinning hair. You shouldn't have to worry about the oil treatment giving your hair a limp, greasy appearance as long as you are using the correct type of oil. The secret to a great hot oil treatment is to find an oil with the right molecular weight. Those with finer hair should opt for a thin oil that is easily absorbed, like coconut oil (Gavazzoni Dias, 2015). Other oils, like sunflower and mineral oils, tend to cling to the hair, giving it a greasy appearance.

Doing Hot Oil Treatments At Home

You don't need to take a special trip to the store for this treatment because your pantry most likely contains the oil you need! Take some plant-based oil (coconut, grapeseed, avocado, hemp seed, olive, or almond) and warm it in a microwave or on the stove. The oil should be warm to the touch but not hot. One way to check if the oil is not too hot is to place a drop or two on your wrist.

Apply the warm oil to the hair and scalp and massage it using your fingertips. Use small circular motions to massage the oil all over the hairline and scalp. When the oil is distributed, use a wide-toothed comb to distribute the product toward the ends of your hair.

Cover the hair with a plastic cap or towel and let it work its magic for 30 minutes. For extra hydration, leave the oil on your hair and scalp overnight. Shampoo and rinse thoroughly. Follow up with conditioner if desired. Don't be alarmed if your scalp needs a second wash to fully remove the oil; this tends to happen if we use a bit too much. If your scalp needs a second wash, don't skip the conditioner.

Hot oil treatments can help moisturize and nourish the hair, making it softer and more manageable. It can also improve hair elasticity, reduce frizz, and enhance the hair's shine.

Moisturizing Techniques

Moisturizing our locks is important for several reasons. Dry hair takes us for a visit to *Brittle Town* and *Dry City* when it's most inconvenient. Moisturizing is key to preventing an unfortunate trip down *Split End Ave*. Moisturizing your hair helps to prevent this by keeping it soft and supple. It also encourages better length retention and gives hair a healthy sheen. That's because moisturized hair reflects the light better and is generally easier to comb and style. It is especially important for people with naturally curly or coily hair textures, as these hair types tend to be drier and require more moisture to maintain their health and appearance. Two popular techniques for moisturizing hair are the LOC method and the use of humectants.

LOC Method

Perhaps you've heard of the LOC method for curly, coily, and textured hair. It's a game-changing technique that focuses on layering your hair products in a specific order to maximize moisture retention. The method is called LOC, which stands for liquid/leave-in, oil, and cream. This will help to keep the scalp happy and healthy. So, here's the breakdown of the LOC method.

- **L:** First, you start with the L, which stands for liquid/leave-in. You need a water-based product to add moisture and open the hair shaft, making it easier for the oil to absorb in the next step.

- **O:** Next up is the O, which stands for oil. In this step, you add mega moisture to your hair with an oil-based product. The oil could be any natural oil, such as coconut oil, jojoba oil, or olive oil (How to Use the LOC Method, n.d.).

- **C:** Finally, you move on to the C, which stands for cream or butter. This last step breathes new life into curls.

So there you have it, the LOC method in a nutshell. The LOC method helps to keep hair moisturized and hydrated for longer periods, reduces breakage, and promotes healthy hair growth. It is an effective technique for those with dry or brittle hair, abuela-approved!

Humectants

Humectants are ingredients that attract and retain moisture from the air. They are commonly used in hair care products to help moisturize and hydrate the hair. These products are particularly beneficial for Latina hair because this hair type is often prone to frizz and is naturally dry and curly. Humectants can help to keep the hair hydrated, soft, and manageable by drawing in and retaining moisture in the hair shaft. This can help to reduce breakage, split ends, and other types of damage that can be caused by dryness. Common humectants include:

- **Glycerin:** A natural humectant that creates a thin layer over the hair strand and attracts moisture from the environment. In order to avoid excessive water absorption, it is important to dilute glycerin before use. Glycerin is highly humectant and can extract water from its surroundings, including the water in your hair. Supercharge your conditioner by adding glycerin in a 1:5 ratio and mixing thoroughly. Apply the mixture to wet hair, leave it on for up to five minutes, and rinse with plain water.

- **Honey:** A natural humectant filled with nutrients that can improve the overall health of the scalp (Honey for Hair: The

Benefits and How to Use It, n.d.). It's the perfect ingredient to use if you want to maintain healthy, soft, and smooth hair. If you're new to using honey on your hair, give these two recipes a try to see how your hair responds.

- **Honey and oil deep conditioner:** Combine a tablespoon of honey and two tablespoons of coconut oil or olive oil. Warm the mixture to make a hot oil treatment and apply warm to the hair and scalp. Cover the hair and allow the honey and oil to work their magic for at least 20 minutes. Shampoo and complete your hair care routine as normal. If you have fine or limp hair, it's advised to combine honey with coconut oil, as other oils may be too heavy.

- **Honey and ACV cleanser:** Combine half a tablespoon of honey with 10 drops of apple cider vinegar and mix well. Apply the mixture to damp hair and allow it to sit for 15 minutes. Rinse with warm water and complete your hair care routine as desired. Honey and apple cider vinegar work together to clarify the hair and scalp, removing product buildup without stripping natural oils. Apple cider vinegar can also add shine by sealing the outer cuticle layer, which helps to retain moisture (Collins-Hermanstein, n.d.).

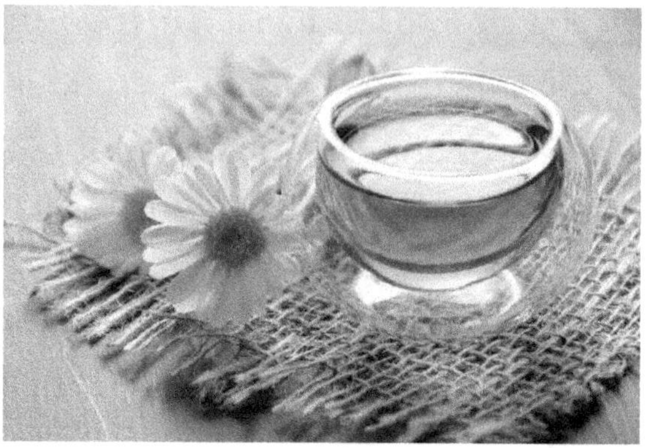

- **Pro vitamin B5:** Also known as D-Panthenol, it can improve hair elasticity by increasing the water content of hair (Panthenol (Pro-Vitamin B5), n.d.). It's commonly used in hair care products and is an effective humectant.

- **Caprylic/capric triglycerides:** Often mistaken for fractionated coconut oil, this humectant imparts a silky feel to hair. Caprylic/capric triglycerides have a dry, silky texture, while fractionated coconut oil feels like a regular carrier oil. As an emollient, it efficiently penetrates the surface to moisturize and condition the hair and provides a lightweight, non-greasy barrier to help retain moisture (Capric Triglyceride in Hair Care Products, n.d.)

- **Aloe vera:** A natural humectant that penetrates the hair, binding water to the hair strand for shiny, hydrated locks. Aloe vera is great to use on the scalp as well. For those with dry scalps, aloe vera can provide nutrients and enzymes to promote hair health. Combining aloe vera and glycerin can add moisture to the hair and improve its vitality. To create a hair mask, mix two to three tablespoons of glycerin with fresh aloe vera gel and apply it to your hair and scalp. Let it sit for 15 to 30 minutes before rinsing it with lukewarm water (Soni, 2022).

When selecting hair care products, it is important to look for those that contain humectants as well as other moisturizing ingredients, such as oils and butters, for hair that's begging to be on the cover of *Vogue México*! Humectants are fabulous to use for all hair types and can keep hair moisturized for days.

Humectants work best when the hair is already damp, as they can attract moisture from the air and help to keep the hair hydrated. They are especially useful in dry climates or during the colder months when the air is drier. However, it is important not to overuse humectants, as they can cause the hair to become too moisturized and prone to breakage. This unfortunate situation can be prevented by following these steps:

- **Choose the right humectant:** There are many different types of humectants, including glycerin, propylene glycol, honey, and aloe vera. Choose one that your hair likes. It may take some experimenting, but that's just more opportunities to pamper ourselves!

- **Use a leave-in conditioner:** Look for a leave-in conditioner that contains humectants, as this will help to keep your hair moisturized throughout the day.

- **Apply humectants to damp hair:** Humectants work best on damp hair, as they help to lock in moisture. After washing your hair, blot it with a towel to remove excess water, then apply a small amount of humectant to your hair, focusing on the ends.

- **Avoid using too much:** While humectants can be great for keeping hair hydrated, using too much can cause your hair to become greasy or weighed down. It's advised to start with a small amount, working your way up if need be.

- **Seal in moisture:** After applying a humectant to your hair, use an oil or butter to seal in the moisture. This will help prevent your hair from drying out and keep it looking shiny and healthy.

Overall, using humectants on hair can be a great way to keep it hydrated and healthy. However, it's important to choose the right products and use them correctly to avoid any unwanted side effects. Knowing how to seal moisture in our hair is a vital part of a healthy hair care routine. Another important aspect is nutrition. From supplements to the importance of a healthy diet, we'll investigate some burning questions in the next chapter.

Five
Nutrition and Latina Hair

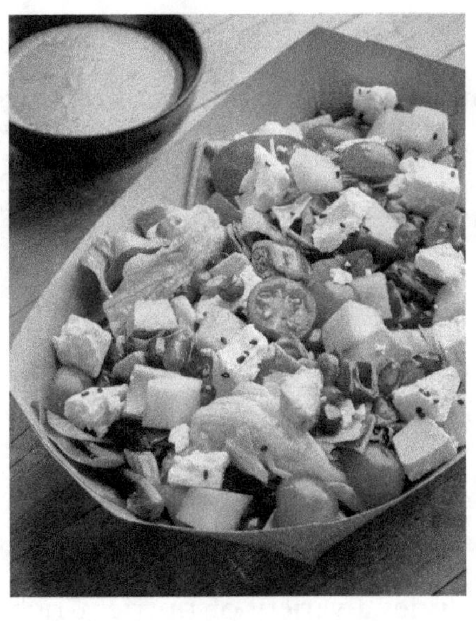

Imagine this: It's dance night. The music is hitting all the right notes, and your hair is behaving—for now, at least. The humidity is high, but you've got faith in the new anti-frizz treatment you're trying. It was formulated for your hair type, so it should do the trick, right? If only it were that straight-forward. Latina hair hair tends to be drier, thicker, and more resis-tant to treatments and products than other hair types. So it's hardly surprising when the anti-frizz or other treatments fail. The shape of the hair shaft has a lot to do with this. Latina hair is typically wider and flatter than that of other hair types, which makes it harder for natural oils to travel from the scalp down the hair shaft (Hair Science

P2: The Hair Types, 2023). As a result, Latina hair can become dry and brittle, which can lead to breakage and split ends.

This is where good nutrition can save the day.

Nutrition is important for hair health because hair follicles require a variety of nutrients to grow and maintain a healthy head of hair. That means our diets should have adequate amounts of protein as well as other vitamins and minerals for our hair to stay healthy. For example, B vitamins such as biotin, niacin, and vitamin B12 are essential for healthy hair growth, while vitamin C is necessary for collagen production, which is an important component of hair structure (Almohanna et al., 2019). Iron, zinc, and omega-3 fatty acids are also important for maintaining healthy hair (Raman, 2022).

Our diets might stray on the carb-rich side, but all those legumes, root veggies, and plantains are great sources of vitamins and minerals. Without adequate nutrition, hair can become weak, brittle, and prone to breakage (Cherney, 2023). Worst of all, your hair may even fall out. We can save ourselves from hair trauma by following a healthy and balanced diet that includes a variety of nutrient-rich foods. Nutrients that are important to the good health of our hair include the following:

- **Protein:** Hair is made up of keratin, so it's important to consume adequate amounts of protein to support healthy hair growth and maintenance (Raman, 2022). Protein is essential for the production of new hair cells, and it also helps to strengthen hair strands. Good sources of protein include lean meats like chicken, fish, and turkey, as well as plant-based sources like beans, lentils, and tofu.

- **Omega-3 fatty acids:** Our bodies can't make omega-3, so it needs to come from our diet. These essential fatty acids are important for maintaining hydration and nourishment in the hair (Petre, 2019). They also help reduce inflammation in the body, which can lead to healthier hair follicles (Hjalmarsdottir, 2023). Good sources of omega-3s include fatty fish like salmon, mackerel, and sardines, as well as nuts and seeds like walnuts and chia seeds.

- **Vitamins A, C, and E:** These vitamins are important for maintaining the strength, elasticity, and hydration of the hair (Davidson, 2021). Vitamin A helps to produce sebum, which is a natural oil that helps to moisturize the scalp and prevent dryness. Hair needs to be protected from free radicals, which is where Vitamin C can help. This vitamin is an antioxidant and helps combat the damage done by free radicals. Vitamin E also has antioxidant properties and helps to improve circulation, which can promote healthy hair growth (SciTechDaily, 2022). Good sources of these vitamins include colorful fruits and vegetables like apricots, peppers, spinach, and tomatoes.

- **Healthy fats:** Olive oil, avocados, and nuts contain healthy fats that can help nourish the hair from the inside out, leaving it shiny and healthy-looking. They also help keep the scalp moisturized, which can prevent dryness and flakiness.

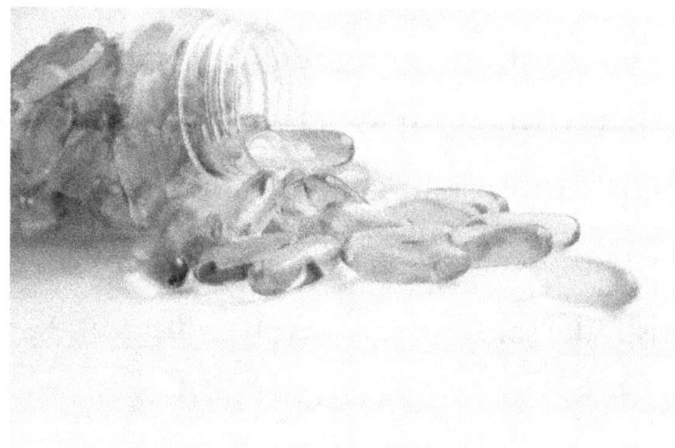

Adequate amounts of protein, omega-3 fatty acids, vitamins A, C, and E, and healthy fats will go a long way toward keeping hair healthy and strong. It's important to drink plenty of water and avoid consuming too much alcohol and sugar, as these can dehydrate the hair and lead to damage (Better Health Channel, n.d.). Bear in mind that hair health is affected by a variety of factors, including genetics, environmental factors, and hair care practices. However, we can give our hair a fighting chance by strengthening it from the inside out.

What You Need to Know About Grays

Two types of pigments are responsible for all the gorgeous hair colors in the world. These pigments are eumelanin (a dark pigment) and pheomelanin (a light pigment). As we grow older, the pigment cells that produce color start to die off. As a result, new hairs growing from the scalp become lighter in appearance, eventually turning gray, silver, and white. When the process has stopped, Follicles won't produce melanin again (Gardener, 2021). Now, we may blame stress, a poor diet, or lifestyle choices for the sudden increase in grays, but in reality, genetics plays a dominant role in determining when our inner silver fox wants to be set free. Chances are, if your parents had a full head of gray hair in their early 40s, then you will too. Of course, race plays a role, too, with the average Caucasian person starting to gray in their mid-30s. Latinas, African Americans, and Asians don't typically see color changes until their early to late 40s (Gardener, 2021).

Sometimes health problems can encourage the formation of gray hair. If we have a shortage of vitamin B12 in our diets, our bodies won't have all the building blocks they need to produce pigment, which could lead to gray hairs. Thyroid disease, vitiligo, alopecia areata, and certain rare, inherited diseases can also encourage the formation of gray hair (Gardener, 2021). Most of the time, though, gray hairs can be traced to nutritional deficiencies, genetics, and lifestyle factors such as stress and smoking.

Stress does not switch off the pigment-producing cells in our skin, but it does cause us to shed at a much faster rate. With increased shedding, there's a bigger chance that the hair that grows back is gray. Smoking is a habit that impacts every single cell in the human body, so naturally, it would encourage gray hairs to take root earlier. It's also a habit that can make silver hair take on a yellow appearance, so you may have to break out the purple shampoo more frequently to combat those brassy tones.

Whatever you do, resist the urge to pluck gray hairs. Plucking won't delay the inevitable, and you may end up damaging the hair follicles so much that hair won't grow from them. Over time, habitual plucking can lead to thin, wispy hair—the exact opposite of what most women want.

Gray hair needs extra love and care. That's because the cuticle is on the thinner side. So don't neglect your sun and heat protection, and try to limit heat styling wherever possible. The thinner cuticle can give gray hair a dry, fragile feel, so we need to ensure that the strands are moisturized and protected. Hair oils and anti-frizz products can help to tame unruly grays, while purple shampoo (a shampoo containing purple pigment) can help to combat brassy yellow tones.

If you only have a few gray hairs and don't feel like committing to a full head of dye, there are a few ways we can camouflage things. A pretty headband, different parts, or a snazzy updo can go a long way to hiding those sneaky strands. Or you could commit to a full head of dye. It's recommended to ask a professional for help. If you are the queen of DIY, look for a product that is designed to cover grays. Permanent color will cover grays better, but it can be a total nightmare to remove if the results are not what you desire. Semi-permanent colors may not cover grays effectively but are generally easier to remove if the results are not as intended. Of course, it is possible to go gray gracefully and ditch the dye. A talented stylist can turn those gray strands into a statement piece, allowing you to rock those locks with confidence.

Supplements to Consider for Healthy Hair

Supplements can help boost the nutrient content of a diet. Supplements can be useful for healthy hair because they provide essential nutrients that may be lacking in the diet. These nutrients are typically delivered in concentrated forms, which are enough to support healthy hair growth and maintenance. However, it's important to note that supplements should not replace a healthy, balanced diet, which should be the body's primary source of nutrients. It's always best to speak to a healthcare professional before taking any supplements or making dietary changes. Here's what to look for:

- **Biotin:** Biotin, also known as vitamin H or B7, is a water-soluble B vitamin that plays a crucial role in maintaining healthy hair, skin, and nails. Biotin deficiency is rare but can cause hair loss, dry skin, and brittle nails (Trüeb, 2016). Researchers found that biotin supplementation can improve the condition of our hair, preventing hair loss in some cases (Patel et al., 2017). Eggs, whole grains, nuts, and leafy greens are some of the foods that are rich in biotin.

- **Vitamin C:** Vitamin C is a water-soluble vitamin that acts as an antioxidant, protecting your hair from damage caused by free radicals. It also plays a key role in the production of collagen, a protein that makes up a significant portion of hair (MedlinePlus, n.d.). Collagen is responsible for maintaining the strength, elasticity, and moisture of hair. Vitamin C deficiency can cause hair breakage and slow hair growth (Julson, 2023). Eating foods rich in vitamin C, such as citrus fruits, berries, kiwis, and peppers, or taking a vitamin C supplement are good ways to keep hair strong.

- **Fish oil:** Fish oil supplements are a rich source of omega-3 fatty acids, which are essential for maintaining hair hydration and preventing hair loss (Frothingham, 2019). Omega-3 fatty acids, particularly EPA and DHA, help to nourish the hair follicles and improve blood circulation to the scalp. In a six-month study, participants who took a fish oil supplement experienced a significant improvement in hair density and thickness (Le Floc'h et al., 2015). Fatty fish, such as salmon, mackerel, and sardines, are also good sources of omega-3 fatty acids.

- **Folic acid:** Also known as vitamin B9, it is essential for healthy hair growth. It helps to produce red blood cells, which deliver oxygen and nutrients to hair follicles (Folate (Folic Acid)—Vitamin B9, n.d.). Without adequate oxygen and nutrients, hair follicles may not function properly. This can result in hair loss and slow hair growth, which can be frustrating. Folic acid deficiency is rare, but it can cause hair thinning and premature graying (Gupta, 2019). Foods rich in folic acid include leafy greens, beans, lentils, and fortified grains.

Giving your hair the nutrition it needs is just one part of a healthy hair care routine. A balanced diet and proper hair care practices, such as gentle shampooing, avoiding heat styling tools, and protecting your hair from the sun and harsh weather conditions, are also essential for maintaining healthy and strong hair. In the next chapter, we'll take a look at the ways we can protect our hair from the elements.

Six

How to Protect Latina Hair From the Sun and the Elements

Have you ever had a neat bun that was ruined by flyaways on a windy day? Sacrificing style just because of the weather can be a bummer, but the right hair tactics can keep your do sleek and stylish no matter what Mother Nature throws at you. Exposure to the sun and other elements can be harmful to hair; that's a no-brainer. But did you know that certain hair types are more prone to damage than others? A lot of our hair woes have to do with moisture, as Latina hair is often thicker and coarser and tends to be drier than other hair types.

All this means is that our hair deserves a little extra care and protection to maintain its health and vitality. As Latinas are no strangers to the sun, that protection (and a bottle of water) will become extra important.

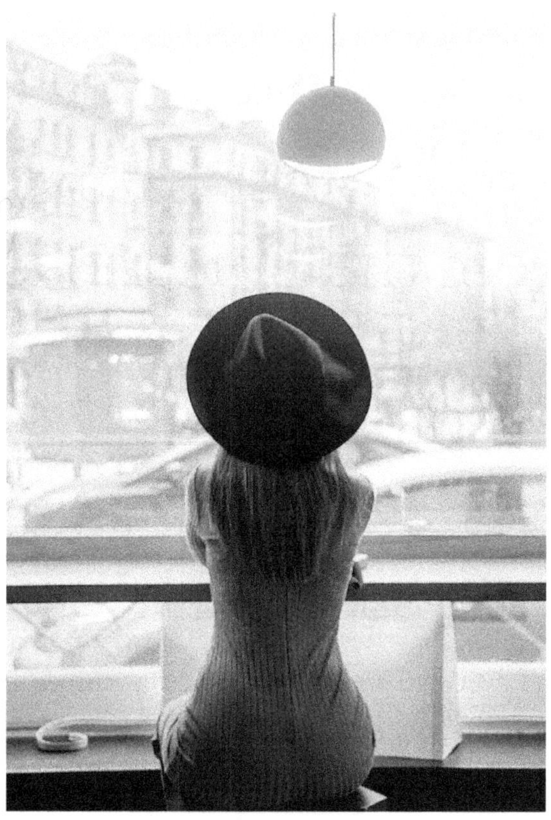

Water is essential for healthy hair. Adequate hydration plays a critical role in various bodily functions, including regulating body temperature, transporting nutrients, lubricating joints, and flushing out toxins. One of the most significant benefits of drinking water is its effect on the skin and hair. Proper hydration helps to keep the skin moisturized, soft, and supple. It can also reduce the appearance of fine lines and wrinkles, as well as prevent skin dryness and flakiness. Similarly, drinking enough water can help keep the hair hydrated and healthy.

Dehydration can cause hair to become brittle and prone to breakage, leading to slower hair growth (Can the Amount of Water You Drink Affect Hair Loss and Growth? n.d.). On the other hand, adequate hydration can help promote healthy hair growth and reduce hair fall. Therefore, it is important to drink enough water to keep your body hydrated, promote healthy skin and hair, and maintain overall health.

Latina Hair and Sun Protection

UV radiation from the sun can cause damage to the hair shaft, leading to dryness, brittleness, and breakage (UV and Your Hair, 2022). That's because UV radiation damages the bonds that hold the hair together. As these bonds break down, keratin is lost, and our hair becomes drier and thinner in the process. That's not all. Environmental pollutants can accumulate in the hair, leading to buildup and further damage. Prolonged sun exposure is one of the reasons why that freshly dyed head of red hair won't maintain its vibrancy for too long either, or why highlights become brassy. The more keratin is lost, the more porous the hair strand becomes, allowing more color to leach when exposed to water. Our hair goes through a lot, so a little protection from the sun and elements can help to keep it healthy.

Sunscreens specially formulated for hair can help provide much-needed protection. These products contain specific protective agents to help prevent damage caused by UV radiation and environmental pollutants. When choosing a sunscreen, select a formulation that is lightweight or it could weigh the hair down.

Hats and Headgear to Protect Hair

In addition to using sunscreen, wearing a hat can be helpful in providing extra shade for your hair. Wide-brimmed hats can be particularly helpful. Cotton or synthetic cotton hats can help keep hair moist and protect it from direct sunlight.

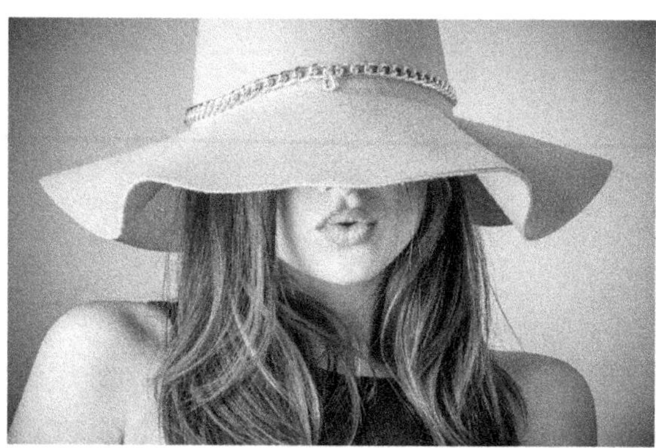

Remember to keep hair well-moisturized by regularly using a deep conditioner or hair mask to maintain health and vitality (Kunin, n.d .). By using sunscreen, wearing a hat, and keeping hair well-moisturized, we can say "goodbye" to flyaways and unruly hair and welcome strong, resilient, and beautiful hair.

Dealing With The Elements

A light breeze can be sexy, but a strong gust of wind can spell disaster if you're not prepared. To start, plan an updo of some sort. Leaving your hair completely down gives the wind free reign to create intricate knots and tangles.

The elements can be a problem too. Rainy and humid weather can turn our gorgeous locks into a frizzy mop. Use an anti-frizz leave-in conditioner after drying, and if you live in a particularly humid or rainy area, use a leave-in treatment that's labeled for daily use. Using a light coat of hairspray or hair gel can also help protect and smooth your hair.

Planning a day outside? Consider how you'd protect your hair. If you're planning to swim, wet your hair before stepping into the pool. The reason for this is simple: We soak our hair with plain tap water to prevent it from absorbing pool water and all the chlorine it contains. You can even add a leave-in conditioner to wet hair before heading out to the beach or pool.

Protective Products for Latina Hair

There are different ways Latinas can protect their gorgeous tresses in addition to the use of sunscreens. Whether you feel like rocking a snazzy hat, sleek headwrap, or a cute protective style, it's recommended to use protective products that contain UV filters to block ultraviolet rays and minimize sun damage. Some of the protective products that are worth using include:

- **Coconut oil:** This hair-loving oil does offer some protection against the sun, blocking an estimated 20% of UV rays (Dixon, 2013). On its own, coconut oil will not offer enough protection, but it can turn those sun-worshiping days into a treat for your hair. If you're spending time at the beach or pool, moisten your curls with some water or leave-in conditioner. Add a thin layer of coconut oil on top, and you've given your hair a moisture boost to fight the drying effects of salt and chlorine.

- **Barriers**: A physical barrier between our hair and the sun is always a fashionable idea. Hats and scarves are good choices when we spend the day outside and give the scalp much-needed protection from the sun. For UV protection, when you're going for a swim, mix two teaspoons of sunscreen in a cup of water and add three or four drops of rosemary oil to a spray bottle (Woodford, 2020). Remember to reapply the mixture as you go in and out of the water.

- **After-sun mask:** If your fun in the great outdoors left your hair feeling fried, it would be a good idea to use a hair repair mask after shampooing. Use a repair mask suited for your hair and scalp type; three to five minutes is usually enough time for it to work its magic. Masks that offer an intense hydrating effect will help restore life to sun-fried locks.

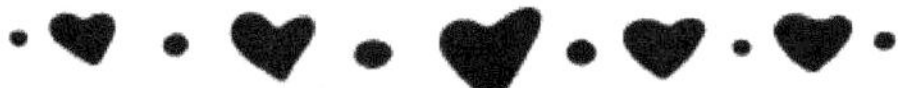

Protective Hairstyles

Rocking a protective hairstyle is a great way to shield your hair from the sun and other environmental elements that can damage it. These types of hairstyles can vary greatly in terms of the amount of manipulation required to install and maintain them. No-manipulation styles, like box braids, don't require much daily attention, while low-manipulation styles, like twists and buns, require some attention every day. Protective hairstyles are recommended for anyone with curly or kinky hair. If your hair is fine or prone to breakage, if you live in a harsh environment, or if you are busy and can't style your hair every day, protective styles can be a lifesaver.

There are some common myths about protective styles. For example, some people think that they're the only or best way to grow your hair, but this is not true. Hair can still grow even when not in a protective style, and the secret to hair growth is care and consistency. Also, not all protective styles are automatically good for your hair. They have to be carefully installed, maintained, and refreshed to avoid causing breakage, hair loss, tangling, and dryness.

It's essential to care for hair that's in protective styles by keeping it moisturized and the scalp clean. It's not recommended to leave the style in for too long. Although protective styles don't cause hair to grow any faster than usual, they can prevent breakage and hair loss that is typically caused by daily or weekly styling. However, if installed improperly or kept in for too long, they can slow down hair growth. It's recommended to keep protective styles for two to three weeks to avoid tangling, dryness, breakage, matting, and buildup of dirt and grease (Myths and Tips about Protective Styles! 2021). That being said, let's take a closer look at some of these protective styles.

Braids

One of the most popular protective hairstyles is braids. Braids can help to protect your hair from the sun's harmful rays by providing a barrier between your hair and the sun. If a loose braid is more your style, those can help, too, as they minimize the amount of pulling and tugging that hair is subjected to when we sleep. This means less breakage and longer hair. Braids can be as intricate as you want them to be, but a rope braid comes together quickly when you get the hang of it. The braid is very easy to learn and only requires two sections. If your bands won't stay in place in most other braids, give rope braids a try. The twists tend to keep things in place, no matter how hot and humid the day becomes. That being said, here's how to do a simple rope braid.

- Brush and part the hair into two sections. Now for the tricky part: twist the sections towards the front of your face. You'll need to maintain a firm grip to keep the section from unraveling in the next step.

- After the sections are twisted, gently cross them over each other. The sections need to cross each other in the opposite direction you twisted. Since we twisted the sections towards the face, we need to cross them away from the face.

- Add small pieces of hair to each twist, twisting the section toward the face and crossing away from the face. Repeat this step to form the braid and secure it with a hair tie.

- Pancake the braid by gently tugging on sections starting from the top. This gives the braid volume.

Twists

Similar to braids, twists can help shield your hair from the sun and reduce breakage. They can also be a great option if you're looking for a low-maintenance hairstyle that can last for several weeks. Twists may be beneficial for hair growth by minimizing the amount of manipulation that the hair is subjected to. The bonus is that they are super easy to do. Rope twists give our hair lovely, tight coils and tend to last longer. Here's how to do it:

- Start with washed and deep-conditioned hair. Part your hair into small sections and apply your preferred leave-in conditioner. Detangle if necessary.

- Split the section into two parts and create a small rope braid. Secure the braid. Repeat with the other sections and style as desired.

- Dry hair overnight for defined, no-heat spiral curls.

Buns

Another protective hairstyle that can help shield your hair from the sun and other elements, buns are a great option if you're looking for a stylish and sophisticated look, all while minimizing the amount of friction our hair is exposed to simply by keeping it in place. That doesn't mean buns have to be boring or require an army of bobby pins to secure. The loop bun is one of those fun hairstyles that complement any occasion.

- Start with a ponytail and divide it into two sections.

- Use one section to create a loop. Take one section of the ponytail and loop it over the other section of the ponytail. Hold the loop in place with your fingers.

- Take the other section of the ponytail and loop it over the first section of the ponytail, creating a second loop. Hold this loop in place with your fingers.

- Once you have created the loops, secure them in place with bobby pins. Make sure to hide the bobby pins so that they are not visible.

- Adjust the loops to make them even and tidy. Slide bobby pins into the hair to secure loose strands. Finish with hairspray to keep it in place.

In addition to these protective hairstyles, there are also several other steps that you can take to help protect your hair from the sun and other elements. For example, wearing a hat or scarf can help shield your hair from the sun's harmful rays. Additionally, using a leave-in conditioner or hair oil can help to moisturize and nourish your hair, which can help to prevent breakage and promote growth.

Sometimes a cute braid or messy bun won't cut it. Knowing which hairstyles are the most flattering on Latina hair can give us that extra shot of confidence when we need it. From chic bobs, edgy pixies, and modern braids to a loose mane with curls, there are many flattering hairstyles that suit Latina hair beautifully.

Seven

The Best Hairstyles for Latina Hair

Latin culture is renowned for its bold and daring fashion choices. Our hairstyles are no exception. Even when we rock long, dyed hair, we showcase our personality and creativity. Whether it's a vibrant shade of red or a bold ombre, dyed hair is a statement-making style that has become increasingly popular in recent years. This look works particularly well on long hair, allowing the color to really pop and draw attention. Whether you choose to dye all of your hair or just add highlights, this is a great way to experiment with color and express your individuality.

Many Latina women dye their hair for various reasons, with blonde being a popular choice. Dirty blonde shades complement Latina complexions well, whether done through highlights or a full-dye job.

In terms of hairstyles, Latinas have come up with many creative ways to style their long hair. A simple ponytail is a no-nonsense option that works well for those who are highly active and need a style that won't get messed up easily. The asymmetrical flow is another popular style that balances fashion and function, with the hair simply taken to one side (Moore, 2022). The middle part is a classic style that works best with extremely long hair, while the textured waves give a more dimensional look that suits shorter hair.

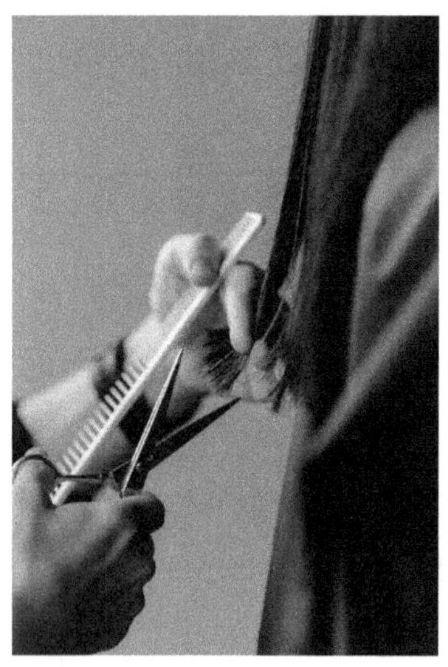

The long bob with subtle side parting is absolutely stunning on Latina hair, but the messy ponytail looks just as good! Waterfall styles add volume and texture to wavy hair, creating a completely different look. These hairstyles are just a few examples of the many styles that Latinas have developed and embraced over time. Remember, Latina hair is diverse and can be straight, wavy, curly, kinky, or any combination of these, so don't be afraid to try out different styles that work best for you!

Hairstyle Considerations

When choosing a hairstyle that's perfect for you, there are a few things to keep in mind. Firstly, you'll want to consider your hair type. It's important to choose a style that works well with your hair type to achieve the best results. For instance, if your hair is naturally straight, you wouldn't want to pick a style that's designed for extremely curly hair.

It's a good idea to decide on the length of your hair first. Short hairstyles can look pretty different from long ones, so it's often easiest to decide on the length of your hair before choosing a style that complements it.

Heritage can be an essential factor for many Latina women when it comes to choosing a hairstyle. If this resonates with you, you may want to consider wearing a style that reflects it.

Hairstyles That Are Always In Vogue

Hairstyles have been an essential aspect of fashion and beauty for centuries. They are ever-evolving, and new trends keep emerging. One of the most fascinating things about hairstyles is that they have the power to transform one's appearance instantly. Latinas are known to showcase hairstyles that are trendy and unique. Whether you have long or short hair, thick or thin, there is a hairstyle that will suit you.

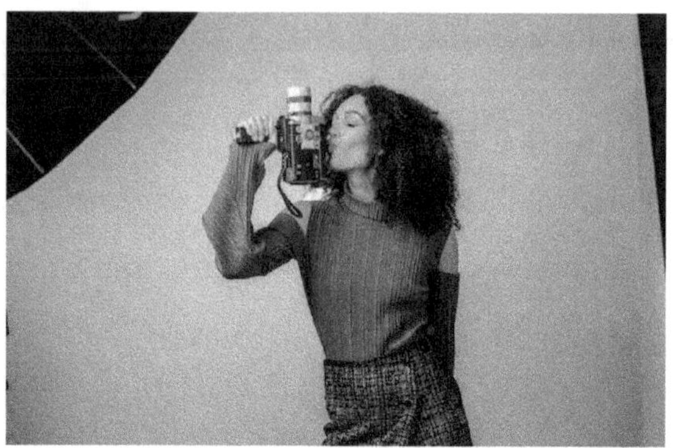

Thick and curly hair is a common trait among Latinas, and it is also one of the most enviable. Curls are moody and come in different textures, but the playful touch they lend to hairstyles makes them enchanting. For those with thick, curly hair, it is best to consider styles that let curls hang free. That being said, some hairstyles are truly evergreen and simply make sense on Latina hair from a fashion perspective.

- **Short bobs:** Short bobs are perfect for those with naturally voluminous hair. The short and stylish haircuts always look ready for a night out. You can rock those curls for a fuller appearance or wispy waves for a playful romance-novel look. If you want to make a statement, a bold pixie cut is the way to go.

- **Braids and bouncy curls:** Many Latinas are blessed with naturally curly hair that can be styled in a number of ways. Bouncy curls and braids are two such styles that accentuate the natural beauty of hair. Braids are versatile and can be dressed up or down or add a new dimension to half-up styles. When curly hair is maintained, it looks simply stunning without extra effort. Shakira has set the standard for gorgeous curls, so if you want to achieve similar curls, you'll need to take care of them every day.

- **Classic pony:** Ponytails are a go-to option for many ladies out there, and Latinas love to rock their ponytails with a curly appearance. This versatile hairstyle can be worn almost everywhere, from a casual day out to a formal event.

- **Top knot:** A top knot is a great choice for every occasion, especially if you are a Latina with naturally curly hair. The style is sleek, voluminous, and suitable for any occasion.

Whether you choose to go with your natural curls or try something new, there are endless possibilities when it comes to hair. So, embrace your hair and experiment with different hairstyles to find the one that suits you the best.

Hairstyles for the Fashionista

Latina hair is truly a gift to the fashion world. Not only do our gorgeous tresses bring out the beauty of many hairstyles, but we are trendsetters! Latina celebrities are often an inspiration for fierce, fun, and stylish haircuts. Puerto Rican model Joan Smalls has been known to rock long layers. It's her secret to create loose waves without them becoming too choppy (Palomares, 2015). Salma Hayek's medium-length hair is often worn naturally curly, giving her an effortless and flawless look. And who can forget Eva Longoria's fun, layered midi cut? It was a refreshing twist on the traditional medium-length cut. Whether you have naturally thick hair or not, there's a perfect hairstyle for you to try. Here are a few ideas:

- **Highlighted perm:** Highlights are breathtaking on dark hair. It should be noted that this hairstyle will require a perm if your hair is not naturally curly. The result is very flattering but hinges on how well we take care of our curls. Experiment with colors to add some flair, and remember to protect and treat the hair as needed to keep follicles hydrated and healthy.

- **Romantic highlighted waves:** One way to make hair runway-ready is to experiment with highlights. Flattering highlights and gentle waves create a classic romantic look that won't go out of style.

- **Waves and side-swept bangs:** Long hair does not mean we can't enjoy bangs! Long, side-swept bangs are perfect for date night, especially when the rest of our hair is styled into neat waves. It's a flattering style that will suit most women with long hair.

- **Thick curls:** This hairstyle requires us to wear our hair in thick and neat curls, creating a sophisticated look. With a few strategic highlights, this hairstyle is virtually guaranteed to turn heads.

- **Colored headband:** Headbands are a woman's cheat code for a fantastic hair day. A simple headband can transform any hairstyle, even if the do is dull. Headbands can give any hairstyle some personality and allow us to play with colors and accessories to complete the look.

- **Bandana look:** This simple, casual look keeps our hair wavy and pinned at the back. Two forehead strands frame the face for an effortless, casual look that will complement most women.

- **Sleek and glittery bun:** Sleek all the hair into a flawless bun. A side part works well here. For extra lift, consider using a sponge bump-up clip and firmly secure the hairstyle with bobby pins. A little finishing spray and this sleek hairstyle is ready. It's ideal for formal events. A few well-chosen and well-placed decorative clips can accentuate this hairstyle quite elegantly!

- **Hair crowns:** Attention-grabbing and versatile, hair crowns can be worn on most occasions. Most hair lengths can be fashioned into a sassy hair crown if enough bobby pins are used, so shorter-haired women can give this hairstyle a try. Start from the forehead and create two braids that meet at the back. Use as many bobby pins as needed to secure the hair. Flowers, ribbons, and decorative clips can be used to hide the ends of the braid and decorate this hairdo.

So whether you're going for a classic look or a more modern style, there's a hairstyle to complement your hair.

Braids for Latina Hair

Braids are a simple and modern way to style our hair. There are many types of braids that you can use to show off your gorgeous tresses, from French braids to fishtail braids. No matter which braid you choose, one of the best things about braids is that they beautify our hair without chemicals. We all know that chemical treatments can damage the hair and scalp, so it's always a good idea to find natural alternatives. Braids not only add style to our hair but can also protect it from damage. If you're not sure which braids to try, don't worry! We've got you covered.

Dutch Braids

Dutch braids are similar to French braids, but they are inverted. They look great on all hair types, but they're especially stunning on thick and curly Latina hair. Dutch braids are easy to master and very versatile. Here's how to do it:

- Brush your hair to remove any tangles. Take a section and divide it into three sections.

- Begin braiding the three sections together, crossing the left section under the middle section and then the right section under the middle section.

- On the next pass, add a small section of hair from the left side of your head to the left section before crossing it under the middle section. Repeat on the right side.

- Continue adding small sections of hair to each side as you braid, making sure to keep the braid close to your scalp. Avoid making the braid too tight as best you can. We don't want it pulling our hair out, but it should sit securely.

- Continue braiding until you reach the nape of your neck, and then finish off with a regular braid.

Fishtail Braids

Fishtail braids are more intricate braids, but they look amazing on Latina hair. They can be worn tight or loose and are a great way to show off your hair's texture. Don't worry! The fishtail is easier to braid than most people think! Here's how you do it:

- Brush your hair to remove any tangles. Split the hair into two sections.

- Cross a small section of hair (from the outside of the left section) over to the inside of the right section.

- Repeat on the other side, taking a small section of hair from the outside of the right section and crossing it over to the inside of the left section. Continue alternating sides and crossing small sections of hair until you reach the end of your hair.

- Secure the braid.

Box Braids

Box braids are a popular protective style for Latina hair. They can be styled in different lengths and sizes, and they're a great way to give your hair a break from heat styling and chemical treatments. Even though box braids take time to do properly, the process of creating the braid is a simple one. Here's how to do it:

- Part hair into small sections. Take one section of hair and divide it into three equal sections.

- Begin braiding the three sections together, crossing the left section under the middle section and then the right section under the middle section. Continue braiding until you reach the end of your hair.

- Secure the braid with an elastic band.

- Repeat with the remaining sections of hair until all of your hair is braided.

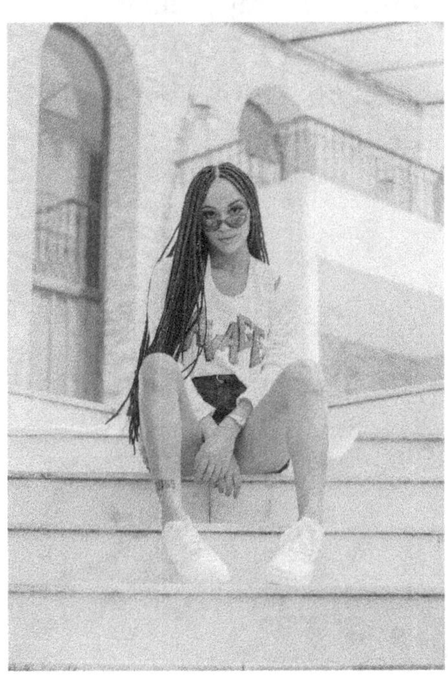

Cornrows

Cornrows are a classic braid style that never goes out of fashion. They can be worn in different patterns and sizes, and they're a great way to keep your hair neat and tidy. Cornrows aren't that difficult to master when you know the steps. Here's what to do:

Create small sections using a comb or your fingers. A rat-tail comb will give us neat, precise sections. Take one section of hair and divide it into three equal sections.

- Begin braiding the three sections together, crossing the left section under the middle section and then the right section under the middle section.

- On the next pass, add a small section of hair to the left section before crossing it under the middle section. Repeat on the right side.

- Continue adding small sections of hair to each side as you braid, making sure to keep the braid close to your scalp. It can be very easy to braid the hair too tightly. The hair should be snug and secure. There shouldn't be any pulling.

- Continue braiding until you reach the end of your hair, and secure the braid with a small hair tie.

There are many other types of braids that you can try, so don't be afraid to experiment with different styles. Just remember to take care of your hair while wearing braids by moisturizing and protecting your scalp.

Hairstyles With Loops

Latina hairstyles with loops are a playful way to switch up your hair game. They can be incorporated into a variety of hairstyles and are perfect for any occasion. Whether you have long or short hair, there are plenty of options to choose from.

- **Fishtail braid with loops:** One of the most popular hairstyles with loops is the fishtail braid with loops. This style combines the intricacy of a fishtail braid with the playfulness of loops. To achieve this look, start by creating a fishtail braid, then use your fingers to gently tug on the loops to make them stand out. You can add as many or as few loops as you like to achieve your desired look.

- **Twisted ponytail with loops:** Another popular hairstyle with loops is the twisted ponytail with loops. This style is perfect for those days when you want to add a little extra flair to a basic ponytail. Start by gently pulling your hair into a low ponytail. Next, divide the ponytail into two equal sections and twist them around each other. Then, create a loop with the twisted hair and secure it with a bobby pin. Repeat this process until you've created as many loops as you like.

- **Box braids with loops:** A popular option for those looking to add a little extra something to their protective style. Section hair into small sections and braid each section into a box braid. Create a small loop at the base of each braid and secure it with a bobby pin. Simple, but cute!

Loops give hairstyles a versatile and modern twist, and there are plenty of ways to make them your own.

Factors to Consider When Selecting a Hairstyle

When it comes to selecting a hairstyle for Latina hair, one of the most important factors to consider is texture. Latina hair can be fine and straight or thick and curly, and the texture of your hair will determine how well a certain hairstyle will work for you. It's important to choose a hairstyle that flatters your natural texture and doesn't require too much manipulation. After all, we want to enjoy our hair.

Face shape is another factor to consider. Different face shapes suit different hairstyles, and choosing a hairstyle that complements your face shape can make a big difference to your looks. While it is possible to wear any style, some hairstyles may flatter your natural features more than others. For example, individuals with round faces may want to opt for a longer hairstyle that elongates the face. Long, shaggy layers are ideal for oval faces, while textured bobs with waves are perfect for all face shapes, including ovals. For square faces, a diamond-shaped haircut or outgrown curtain-style bangs look stunning (Derrick, 2021).

The six main face shapes are oval, square, round, heart, oblong/rectangle, and diamond. The determining factors for face shape are usually the forehead, cheekbones, and jawline.

- An oval face shape is considered the most desirable because its length is greater than its width, with the forehead being the widest part of the face. Almost any haircut flatters this face shape, from long layers to shoulder-length waves, full fringe, layered bobs, or a side-swept pixie.

- A square face shape has a length-to-width ratio that is almost equal, with a strong angled jaw and minimal curve at the chin. To soften the edges around the forehead and strong jawlines, consider wavy shags with a wispy fringe, soft side-swept bangs, or long layers with a fringe. An asymmetrical fringe or softer angles are also excellent options for this face shape.

- A round face shape has a length and width ratio that is about equal, with soft and rounded features, flatter cheekbones, and the cheeks standing out as the widest part of the face. Similar to a square face shape with softer angles, a long bob works well for this face shape as it visually lengthens the face. Long straight hair, long voluminous waves, shaggy bobs, and swoopy bangs with cropped sides also complement this face shape (Derrick, 2022).

- A heart-shaped face has a pointed chin with a wider forehead, usually in the shape of an inverted triangle. Blunt bangs and wavy layers or a chin-length bob with bangs look best, with soft angles in the front that start below the face to balance out the longer forehead. Keeping the bangs narrow creates the illusion of less width at the top.

- An oblong/rectangle face shape has the forehead, cheeks, and jawline at nearly the same width, or the distance from forehead to chin is slightly longer than the distance from ear to ear. Long layers add a dimension of movement and playfulness to the hair and pair beautifully with side-swept or feathered fringes.

- A diamond face shape is usually defined by high cheekbones, a pointy chin, and a narrower forehead. Short-cropped hair shows off the high cheekbones, and keeping it long with face-framing layers is also flattering. Long bangs that caress the cheekbone can serve to accentuate this shape.

Overall, while there isn't always one definitive way to go when selecting a haircut, there are a few flattering and standard tips to accentuate features and create balance. Remember, breaking the rules is allowed, so feel free to experiment until you find the perfect cut for you.

Your lifestyle can also play a role in selecting a hairstyle. If you have a busy schedule or work in a professional setting, you may prefer a low-maintenance hairstyle that can be styled quickly and easily. On the other hand, if you have more free time or prefer a more dramatic look, you may choose a more intricate hairstyle that requires more time and effort to maintain. Of course, personal style is the most important factor in selecting a hairstyle. Whether you prefer a more edgy or classic look, there are a wide range of hairstyles to choose from that can help you express your style. Whatever style you end up choosing, it's always a good idea to arm yourself with tips to keep your hair shiny and healthy.

Eight

Tips to Keep Latina Hair Shiny and Healthy

Some hair care tips just make a lot of sense. If you get your curls cut, make sure that's done on dry hair to enhance the volume and texture of the hairstyle (La Jeunesse, 2020). Latinas rocking straight hair are all too familiar with the battle of flat hair. To prevent the "flatness" from ruining a stunning look, use a volumizing shampoo and conditioner, and apply oil to the ends while styling. Do not apply a non-volumizing conditioner directly to the roots, and avoid choppy haircuts to accentuate the hair's natural beauty. Haircuts with subtle, blended-in layers add more movement and give us plenty of styling options. To maximize volume, rough-dry the hair. Do this by flipping your hair upside down and lifting the roots with your fingers.

Wavy hair doesn't have a volume problem, but it does get weighted down fairly easily. For this reason, lightweight hydrating products can be a game changer. It's also advisable to use a hair mask once every other week and opt for haircuts with shorter blended layers to add fullness and movement. The layers should ideally not be shorter than the chin, depending on hair length and preferences, and complement most faces beautifully.

When it comes to getting the best out of curly hair, your best bet lies with products designated for curly hair. It's preferable to wash hair once or twice a week and comb it while it's still wet. Moisturize hair once a week with a hair mask that has natural ingredients, and try to avoid or minimize the use of products containing alcohol, mousse, gel, and hairspray as they can be drying (Gómez, 2017). As you see, different hair types have different care needs, but some general hair care tips do apply to everyone.

General Care Tips For Lush Hair

In order to keep your hair looking shiny and healthy, it's important to follow a few simple tips. Firstly and most importantly, know your hair type. Start by finding your curl pattern and hair type, and use products suitable for your hair type. Using the right products for your hair type will already make a noticeable difference, and these tips will up your hair game further:

- Deep shampoo once a week to remove any accumulation of products and dirt from your hair. Additionally, use a deep conditioner to keep your hair hydrated and nourished.

- Use moisturizing hair care products to feed your hair to keep your waves or curls hydrated and prevent dryness, knots, and tangles.

- In order to get the most out of protein treatments, it is best to pair them with moisturizing treatments. Doing so will prevent overuse of protein treatments, which can leave hair feeling stiff otherwise.

- For hair to flourish, it is essential that the scalp remains healthy. Co-washing is fantastic for keeping curls clean and hydrated, but it doesn't help the scalp much. Be sure to lather up at least twice a fortnight to remove oil and product buildup from the scalp.

- Maintaining your ends' freshness through cuts is essential for healthy-looking curls. Use wide-tooth combs instead of ordinary hair brushes to avoid damaging those delicate strands.

- Avoid excessive use of hair dryers, irons, and curling irons, as they can cause heat damage to your hair. Additionally, try to avoid using products that contain alcohol, as this can dry out your hair and cause damage.

Don't forget to protect your hair from the sun, either. Try using a sunscreen specifically designed for your hair to keep it looking healthy and shiny.

Hair Washing Mistakes Every Latina Makes

When it comes to washing hair, it may seem like a straightforward task, but there are many pitfalls to avoid to maintain healthy, shiny hair. Washing hair is not just about lathering and conditioning; it involves a shower routine. Improper washing techniques may lead to greasy roots, flat hair, and faded hair color (Pai, 2016). All that money spent at the salon was wasted, thanks to hair-washing mistakes.

Not Soaking Hair

A big mistake that people make is not soaking their hair well with water. Quick head dunks may not be enough to get the hair thoroughly soaked through. The shampoo won't lather up and cleanse the hair well without enough water. So take the time to ensure that the hair is wet before applying shampoo.

Scalding Water

Another mistake is using water that is too hot. Our cuticles open with hot water, allowing keratin, color molecules, and moisture to escape. This can lead to hair becoming dry and color fading. Cooler water helps keep the cuticle sealed, preventing frizz and fading of color.

Excessive Scrubbing

Scrubbing your scalp too vigorously can do more harm than good. If you love a good scalp massage, it's best to go for a gentle approach. Wet hair is weak and prone to breakage, so it is recommended to be gentle while washing your hair. Stroke your scalp gently instead of rubbing it aggressively. Over-scrubbing the scalp can cause the scalp to overproduce oil, leading to greasy roots.

Shampooing Everything

Shampoo is a cleanser, so it should only be applied to areas that get dirty and grimy, mainly the roots. Conditioner belongs to the drier areas of the hair, that is, the mid-lengths of the hair to the ends. Applying conditioner to the roots may weigh the hair down and cause a loss of volume. Skipping conditioner is another mistake. Conditioner gives hair slip and silkiness, reducing friction and protecting it from breakage when brushing or styling it. After cleansing, the scalp regains its natural oils, but the ends remain susceptible to drying out, which is why a conditioner is essential. To apply conditioner, start with the ends, then spread it up to the mid-shaft.

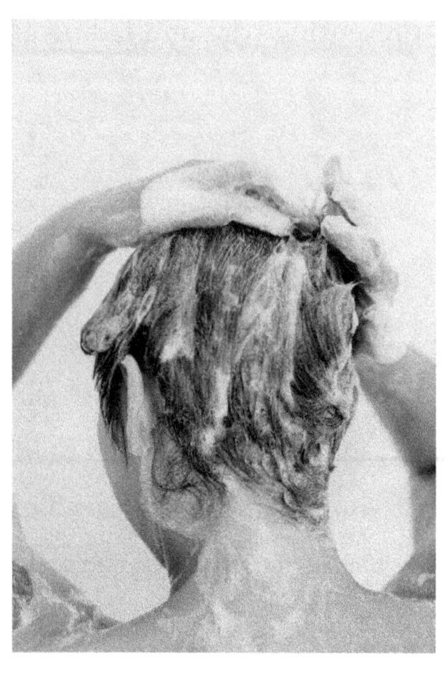

Rushing

Using a shampoo with sulfates is not recommended for those who color their hair. Sulfate-free shampoos are gentler, keep the cuticle tighter, and prevent color fading quickly. Also, rushing through the hair-washing routine is a mistake we all are guilty of from time to time. How many times have we over-shampooed our hair when we are in a hurry? It's easy to forget to rinse the shampoo out of the scalp correctly, which can lead to a number of hair-related problems. Ladies, you know we tend to overuse shampoo, so paying extra attention to rinsing it out of the scalp is a good idea. It is essential to take time to wash hair correctly, especially if the hair is prone to oiliness or dryness.

Hair Wash Routine: A Step-by-Step Tutorial

If you have Latina hair, you may already know that it requires special care to keep it looking its best. This step-by-step guide is put together to help you achieve healthy, shiny hair. Having a proper hair wash routine can save us a lot of hair woes! So without further ado, here's the framework for how to keep hair clean without causing extra damage.

- **Step One:** Use a mild shampoo with neutral pH to clean the hair. Choose a shampoo that is specifically formulated for Latina hair or one that is gentle and free from harsh chemicals. Look for a shampoo with a neutral pH, as this will help to maintain the natural balance of your hair and scalp.

- **Step Two:** Rinse the hair with warm water to open the cuticles and allow deep cleaning. Before applying the shampoo, rinse your hair with warm water to open the cuticles and allow the shampoo to penetrate deeply. We should avoid using hot or scalding water. Hot water will strip natural oils from the hair, encouraging dryness and exacerbating damage.

- **Step Three:** Gently massage the shampoo into the scalp and ends. Apply a small amount of shampoo to your hair, focusing on the scalp and roots. Gently massage the shampoo into your scalp using your fingertips, being careful not to tangle or pull your hair. Work the shampoo down to the ends, but avoid rubbing the hair too vigorously.

- **Step Four:** After shampooing, rinse your hair thoroughly with plenty of water to remove all residues. Make sure to rinse your hair completely, as leftover shampoo can cause buildup and make your hair look dull and lifeless.

- **Step Five:** Use a deep conditioner after shampooing to keep your hair hydrated and healthy. Choose a conditioner that is designed for your hair type and apply it evenly throughout your hair, focusing on the ends. Allow the conditioner to sit on your hair. It needs a few minutes to work its magic before you rinse it out with cool water.

- **Step Six:** Apply a moisturizing or nourishing mask once a week. For an extra boost of hydration and nourishment, use a moisturizing or nourishing hair mask once a week. Apply the mask to your hair and leave it on for the recommended time before rinsing it out with cool water.

By following these simple steps, you can keep your hair looking its best and avoid common hair problems like dryness, breakage, and split ends.

Haircuts Made for Latina Hair

With hair that is diverse in texture and thickness, it can be tricky to find the right haircut that works well for a given hair type. Choosing the right haircut can help manage and enhance the natural features of Latina hair. Considering your hair type, you might consider these cuts:

- **Short and layered haircuts for fine and straight hair:** Latina hair that is fine and straight can benefit from short and layered haircuts. These haircuts add texture and volume to the hair, making it look fuller and more voluminous. Layered haircuts also provide a modern and stylish look to the hair. Layered haircuts with choppy ends create the illusion of thickness and volume, making them a great choice for fine-haired women.

- **Short haircuts with bangs for wavy and thick hair:** Latina hair that is wavy and thick can rock short haircuts with bangs with confidence. These haircuts help manage the hair by providing a defined shape and structure. Short haircuts with bangs work well with wavy and thick hair, creating a polished look.

- **Long haircuts with layers for fine hair:** Long haircuts with layers are a great option for Latina hair that is fine. Layers add volume and texture to the hair, creating a fuller and more voluminous look. Long layers that start at the chin are perfect for helping create the illusion of thickness and volume.

- **Long haircuts with bangs for a modern look:** Long haircuts with bangs look great on hair that is straight or wavy. These haircuts provide a modern and stylish look while also adding structure and shape to the hair. Long haircuts with bangs work well because they help frame the face and create a more polished look.

- **Medium haircuts with a middle part for wavy hair:** This haircut helps manage wavy hair by creating a defined shape and structure. Medium haircuts with a middle part work well with wavy hair because they help create a more balanced and symmetrical look.

- **Bob haircuts for straight and fine hair:** Bob haircuts are a classic option for Latina hair that is straight and fine. This haircut provides a defined shape and structure to the hair, creating a sleek and polished look. Bob haircuts work well with straight and fine hair because they help create the illusion of thickness and volume.

Choosing the right haircut for Latina hair is important to manage and enhance the natural features of the hair. The appropriate haircut will depend on the hair type, texture, thickness, and personal preferences, of course. It is recommended to consult with a professional hairstylist when you feel the need for a dramatic change.

Hair Conditioner Products for Latina Hair

It's no surprise that there has been a surge in beauty brands owned by Latina entrepreneurs. It's a welcome change. As a culture, we have a strong connection to beauty, but many mainstream brands don't cater to our unique needs, particularly when it comes to natural, curly hair. This lack of representation and service in the beauty industry has inspired entrepreneurs to create brands that authentically represent our culture and meet our beauty needs. After years of feeling underserved in the beauty aisles, we have products that understand our hair.

One important tip for maintaining healthy Latina hair is to use a deep conditioner regularly. Deep conditioners contain more concentrated ingredients that penetrate the hair shaft and provide intense hydration (De Bellefonds, 2021). This is especially important for curly hair, which tends to be drier due to its natural shape. Deep conditioners should be used at least once a week for best results.

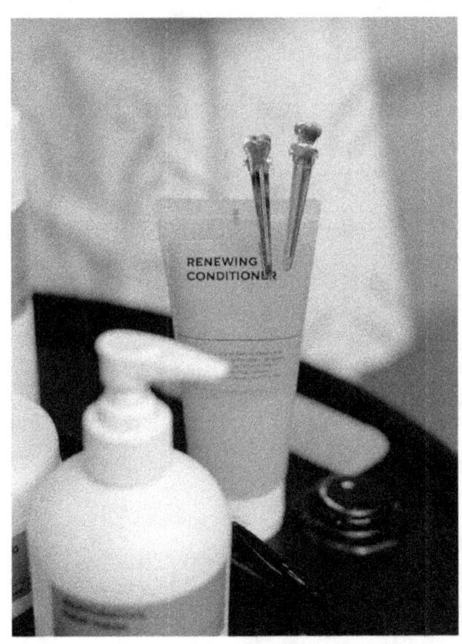

Using Deep Conditioner the Right Way

Deep conditioning helps improve dry and lackluster tresses, making them shinier, healthier-looking, and more resilient. However, it's important to choose the right deep conditioner that suits your hair type. A basic rule of thumb is to opt for a heavier and creamier conditioner if you have thick and coarse hair. Conversely, if you have thin or fine strands, opt for a product that's lighter in texture. To get the most out of your deep conditioning routine, keep the following in mind:

- Read the product labels to understand the claims and how

to use the product correctly. It's also important to avoid over-conditioning, as leaving a conditioning product on the hair for longer than specified can have undesirable results.

- Focus on the mid-length to the ends of your hair when applying a deep conditioner, and avoid applying too much to the roots and scalp. It's easy to overapply a product when it makes our hair feel silky smooth, but using too much can cause greasiness and product buildup.

- Deep conditioning treatments can be done every seven to ten days for those with healthy hair and every three to five days for those with damaged hair that needs more attention (Amra, 2016). It's best to apply a deep conditioner right after washing your hair with shampoo to maximize its benefits. Some deep conditioning treatments also come in the form of hot oils that can help nourish and strengthen hair while protecting against breakage.

Using Suitable Products for Your Hair

Using products specifically designed for Latina hair can change your hair game. These products are often formulated with ingredients that cater to the unique needs of Latina hair. This is why you'll find that many Latina hair products contain natural oils, like argan oil, which can help nourish and hydrate the hair.

It's also important to protect your hair from the sun, especially during the summer months when UV rays can be particularly strong. Using a sunscreen conditioner can help shield your hair from damage and keep it looking healthy.

Natural oils are also great for keeping hair healthy and shiny. Some popular oils include coconut oil, jojoba oil, and castor oil. These oils can be used as a pre-shampoo treatment, a leave-in conditioner, or even as a styling product. These oils can help moisturize hair and reduce frizz.

In addition to regular deep conditioning, it's a good idea to use a moisturizing or nourishing mask once a week to give your hair an extra boost of hydration (Benefits of Using Hair Masks: How Does It Help Your Hair? 2022). When using heat styling tools like hair dryers, irons, and curling irons, it's important to apply conditioning products beforehand to protect the hair from heat damage. Heat-protectant sprays and creams can help prevent breakage and keep your hair looking healthy. These are all important steps we can take to maintain healthy hair. We'll discuss this topic more in-depth in the next chapter.

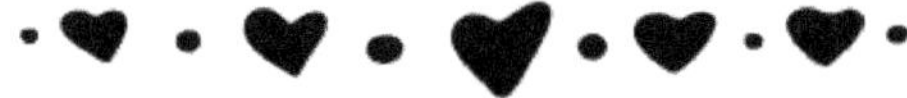

Nine

Maintaining Healthy Hair

There's no denying that a healthy, shiny mane is a confidence boost! Whether we're flaunting a sophisticated bob or playful curls, healthy hair brings out the best in any hairstyle. Naturally, washing our hair is a vital step to ensure that the scalp and hair remain healthy. As much as we love our hair, it is possible to wash it too much. Generally, we should wash our hair when it feels unclean when touched. Washing too frequently strips the hair and scalp of their natural oils, creating an environment for hair problems. Nobody wants oily hair, but all oil isn't bad. The trick is to maintain the right balance on your scalp.

If it were up to shampoo commercials, we'd all be lathering it up every day. In fact, washing our hair too frequently can be the starring cause of many a bad hair day. That's because hair tends to become dry and coarse when free of natural oil. This makes hair notably difficult to style and frizzy. Frizzy hair is never a good look, and Latinas know the struggle all too well. So it should come as no surprise that the driving force behind anti-frizz products was reportedly a Latina (Gonzalez,

2014). Using the appropriate anti-frizz products for your hair type can help improve the manageability of your hair, but we shouldn't over-shampoo our hair.

Many people use an astringent shampoo daily to cleanse their hair. All of this cleaning leaves us with brittle and easily damaged strands. So how often do we need to wash our hair? Maybe not as often as you think. While most of us don't need to wash our hair on a daily basis, how often you lather up will depend on a number of factors, including:

- **Oil:** Oily hair is often considered dirty and can leave hair with an unflattering limp and clumpy look. How much oil we produce is dependent on our age, genetics, environment, and other factors. As we age, the scalp tends to become drier, so we'll need to adapt to its changing needs.

- **Hair type:** Straight and fine hair should be washed more frequently than curly, wavy, or coily hair types. That's because straight hair is more easily coated by the natural oils that our scalp produces, so it will look and feel greasier faster. These oils have a harder time coating thick, coarse, coily, curly, and wavy hair, so it is important not to wash them off too frequently. Sebum is an important part of keeping curls beautiful and well-defined. Most people with tight curls or textured hair types will find that they only need to wash their hair once a week (American Academy of Dermatology, n.d.-a).

- **Sweat:** It's not breaking news that an intense workout can mess up a do, but how much we sweat plays a role in how frequently we'll need to wash or rinse our hair. Sweat can give our hair a dirty feel and look because it helps to spread sebum and can give our hair an unappealing smell. For fresh hair, shampoo after an intense workout or when you wear a hat or helmet for an extended period of time.

- **Pollen, dirt, and debris:** Messy tasks such as gardening and cleaning may stir up dust, pollen, and particles that get stuck in our hair. This debris can give hair a dull appearance and, in some cases, exacerbate allergies. It's best to shampoo your hair after a messy job to keep it feeling and looking clean.

- **Products:** Styling products can leave a residue on the hair and scalp. This buildup can lead to irritation and damage, and frequent product use (or using heavy products) may mean that we need to wash our hair more frequently.

Dandruff is one of the signs that we may be overwashing our hair. Dry hair, an itchy scalp, and flaking all point to an overly dry scalp (Weimert, 2020). A dry shampoo can help refresh our roots and delay wash days, but we should not rely on it too frequently. Occasional use won't harm our hair, but frequent use of dry shampoo can lead to breakage. It's recommended to limit the use of dry shampoo to one or two days a week to keep the scalp and hair healthy (Stanborough, 2019-a). Looking for a natural alternative to dry shampoo? Create this effective dry shampoo powder by using pantry ingredients. You'll need the following:

- ¾ cup cornstarch

- ½ tbsp baking soda

- ¼ cup cocoa powder; use more for darker hair colors (Hill, n.d.)

- 10 drops of essential oil of your choice

Add all the ingredients to a glass bowl and whisk until the mixture is lump free. Store in an airtight glass container and use a broad makeup brush to apply to the roots as needed.

Tight Hairstyles

Another haircare mistake people make is wearing their hairstyles tight. Tight hairstyles can cause damage to your hair in various ways. When you wear tight hairstyles such as braids, cornrows, or tight ponytails, you are putting a lot of tension on your hair. This tension can cause breakage, leading to hair loss and a thinning hairline. Additionally, wearing these styles for extended periods can cause traction alopecia, which is a form of hair loss caused by prolonged tension on the hair (Smith, 2018). Fortunately, there are some changes you can make to your hairstyling routine to help prevent this problem.

First, it's important to avoid frequently wearing hairstyles that pull on your hair. Hairstyles that constantly pull on your hair include tightly pulled buns, ponytails, up-dos, cornrows, dreadlocks, hair extensions or weaves, and tightly braided hair. If you have a habit of wearing rollers to bed, you may be encouraging hair loss as well. Rollers can place quite a bit of tension on the roots of our hair and, if removed incorrectly, can rip it out. Instead, try to wear looser hairstyles that don't put as much tension on your hair.

Loosen your braids, especially around the hairline, to reduce any pulling. Personalize your braids by wearing them thicker, or opt for a braided style that will last for weeks. When choosing a lasting braided style, try to wear the hairstyle for no longer than two months. Hair needs a break from braids too! You should also change up your hairstyle occasionally to reduce the pull, giving your hair a chance to recover. Additionally, you should wear extensions for short periods of time and remove them immediately if they cause pain or irritation.

Lastly, it's important to look for early signs of hair loss, such as broken hairs around your forehead, a receding hairline, or patches of hair loss where your hair is pulled tightly. If you notice any of these signs, it's time to stop pulling on your hair and allow it to regrow (American Academy of Dermatology, n.d.-b). It's also important to change your hairstyle immediately if you experience pain, stinging on your scalp, crusts on your scalp, or tenting (sections of your scalp being pulled up like a tent). By making small changes to our hair routine, we are able to enjoy our sense of style without losing any hair over it.

Hair Care Do's

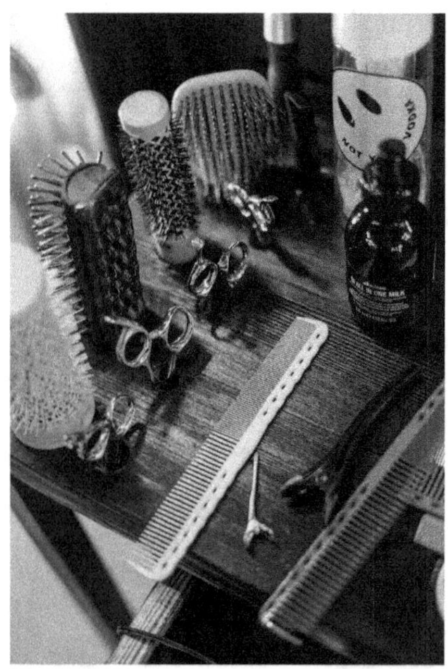

There are many things we can do to maintain our hair. Following a healthy diet, avoiding excessive use of silicon-based products, and refraining from the overuse of hot tools are all excellent ways of ensuring hair health. Another often overlooked aspect of hair health is our brushes.

When it comes to brushes, straight-haired Latinas have it easy. Unless you are dealing with a horde of unruly knots, most paddle brushes work well with straight hair. Hair types with a natural bounce aren't as lucky and will need a brush that is designed to deal with curls. Brushes are designed with different jobs in mind but can be divided into these categories:

- **Comb:** These are used for detangling and sectioning hair.

- **Wet brush:** These are used in or out of the shower. These brushes have flexible bristles to minimize pulling on hair.

- **Boar bristle brush:** Brushes made from boar hair work well on all hair types, especially curly hair. These brushes are ideal for smoothing frizz, distributing oils, and adding shine (Guerra, 2022).

- **Paddle brush:** It's a good brush to use when detangling curly hair and is intended for use on dry hair.

- **Straightening brush:** This intuitive tool straightens hair as you are brushing. It's a gentle method of straightening the hair without the tugs and snags that can happen with flat irons. You'll still need to dry your hair before using a straightening brush and apply heat protectant (Felton, 2020).

- **Hairdryer brush:** A tool that is a combination of a hairdryer and a round brush. It makes a blowout easy to achieve, but heat protectant spray is a non-negotiable before use.

When shopping for a brush, pay attention to the bristles. You'll want to go for a brush that has gentle and flexible bristles. This is to reduce tugging on your hair when brushing. Boar-bristle brushes are a good option, but if you are going for a brush with plastic or nylon bristles, be on the lookout for one with rounded tips. Rounded tips won't scratch the scalp or cause breakage when brushing.

Another thing we need to consider is the brush size. Are you using a big enough brush for the job? For at-home blowouts, it is best to use bigger paddle brushes for straighter and more voluminous hair. Smaller brushes are useful for creating hair full of movement and body. Rocking those natural curls instead? A good wet brush used in the shower with conditioner can make detangling a breeze.

Brushing and detangling your hair can cause breakage and damage. Use a wide-tooth comb or a detangling brush to gently detangle your hair, starting from the ends and working your way up. If you've got knots, the best place to detangle them may be in the shower. Apply conditioner to damp hair, grab the wet brush, and gently run the bristles through your hair to detangle. If your hair is still tangled, consider applying a hair oil or using a detangling spray.

Tips To Prevent Breakage

A regular trim every six to eight weeks is needed when we want to maintain the length and style of a particular haircut. If you're more interested in growing out your locks, it would be best to get a trim every eight to ten weeks to keep split ends in check (The Health Journal, n.d.).

If you're looking to prevent breakage and keep your hair healthy, there are a few things you can do to help maintain its strength and length. Be gentle with your hair. Avoid pulling, tugging, or yanking on your hair, as this can cause damage and lead to breakage. When drying your hair, it's best to gently pat it with a microfiber towel instead of vigorously rubbing it. This helps keep damage to an absolute minimum.

Another tip to prevent breakage is to avoid tight hairstyles. Tight hairstyles like braids, cornrows, or tight ponytails can cause tension and breakage, leading to hair loss. Instead, try wearing looser hairstyles to prevent damage and keep your hair healthy.

When it comes to choosing the right tools for your hair, it's important to use brushes and combs that are gentle and won't cause breakage. A wide-tooth comb is best for detangling. Be gentle when detangling, and use a leave-in conditioner to give your hair extra slip where needed. It's best to avoid using any brushes that have hard bristles, as these can pull the hair and scratch the scalp.

Applying Product Correctly

Hair products can help us set those trendy styles that will become fashion staples for years to come, but if we're not sure how to use our products, we may be damaging our hair. Using hair products the right way is a breeze when you keep these tips in mind.

Small Amounts of Product Works Best

To avoid heavy hair, we need to consider our hair length when using products. Short, sexy pixie cuts require a lot less product than intricate hairstyles, so we need to keep these length differences in mind. A good way to think of product amounts is to describe them in coin sizes. Usually, a dime-sized amount of product is enough for short hair, while a nickel-sized amount serves medium hair well. Long hairstyles may need a quarter-sized amount of product or more to achieve the desired effect.

Use Products on Damp Hair and Comb Through

The difference between "damp" and "wet" is not insignificant. Applying products to wet hair is simply wasteful, as we'll use a good chunk of them as the hair is drying. Allow your hair to dry about 80% of the way before using pomades, mousses, and other products for the best results. If you're curly or wavy-haired, gently scrunch your curls in a towel. Scrunching reduces frizz, especially when a microfiber towel is used. If you're in a hurry and need to get your hair dry quickly, try using a diffuser.

After applying the product, it's always a good idea to gently comb through the hair using a wide-toothed comb. This helps distribute the product evenly for better results.

Volumizers for the Crown and Roots

Some hair products should be used with a specific goal in mind. Volumizers are best used on areas that will give us the most lift (such as the crown and roots). Applying a volumizer anywhere else can leave hair feeling limp and heavy, so it's important to use products as intended.

Massage Mousses

Using a gel, mousse, pomade, or foam? It might be best to massage these products into the hair before drying. This helps coat the hair evenly, increasing the efficacy of the product. When using a pomade or molding paste to texturize sassy, short hair, don't forget to warm a dime-sized amount of the product in your hands before applying it.

Start at the Back

When using a styling product, most people instinctively start to apply it at the top of their heads. This is not very effective, though. If we start applying products from the back of the head, where the hair is thickest, and work our way to the top, we will apply our hair products more efficiently (How to Properly Apply Your Hair Product, 2019).

Every Latina should know that their hair deserves just as much love and care as their skin does. Stepping up your hair game doesn't have to uproot your entire beauty routine. Not at all. In the next chapter, we'll take a look at what it takes to start a basic hair care routine to combat frizz for manageable and shiny hair.

Ten

Embracing Your Hair

Latinas have a very complicated relationship with their hair. Even though beauty outlets and magazines have seemingly unanimously declared that natural hair is trendy, for many Latinas, embracing their curls and kinks amounts to more than just following a trend. For these Latinas, it is about embracing a statement of identity, but to understand this sentiment, we need to keep in mind that hair is more than strands of keratin growing from your scalp. Whether we like it or not, hair brings with it a horde of meaning that is filtered through the cultural lenses through which we view the world. Thankfully, the rhetoric is changing, and Latinas are starting to realize that all hair is *pelo bueno*!

Just because your hair has a different texture does not make it undesirable. All this means is that your hair wants to be treated differently. There are many ways to manage hair, as we've discovered so far. From using the correct products designed for your hair type to using the right hairbrush, we can treat our hair with the love it deserves. Doing so certainly pays dividends, as these Latina stars proved when they flaunted their hair and heritage in public.

- **Amara La Negra:** Sometimes hair becomes the basis of discrimination. It's something that Amara is quite familiar with, as she's dealt with many racial comments about her hair during her career. Like a breath of fresh air, the star made it clear that embracing her natural hair did not detract from her talent (Wright, 2022).

- **Camila Alves:** The Brazilian model certainly knows how to flaunt her dreamy waves, but there was a time when heat and chemical treatments constituted a large part of her haircare routine. Having had enough of hair that was becoming finer and thinner, Alves embraced her natural texture and seemingly never looked back.

- **Stephanie Beatriz:** This actress usually flaunts her gloriously wild curls, whether she's voicing Mirabel Madrigal in *Encanto* or playing a badass detective on the small screen.

Celebrities are usually the culprits behind setting unrealistic beauty standards. That's why it is so refreshing to see these chicas (and others) proudly rocking their natural hair. On or off the screen, well-groomed hair is beautiful. A hair care routine will take the guess-work out of hair care, leaving you more time to enjoy your hair.

Developing a Hair Care Routine

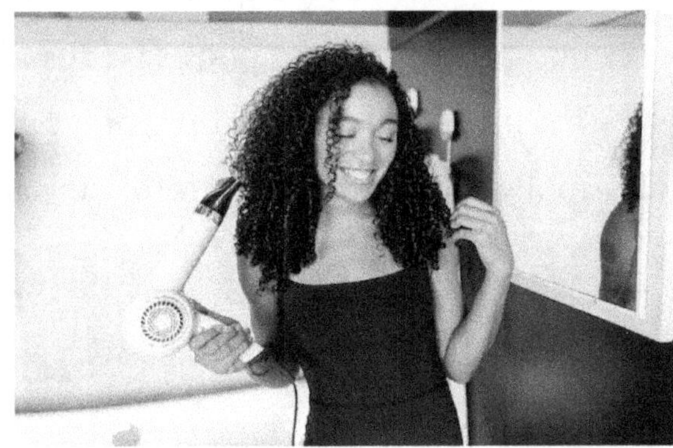

Developing a hair care routine is important for maintaining healthy hair. This routine should include washing your hair with a gentle shampoo and conditioner that are appropriate for your hair type. It's also important to use a deep conditioning treatment once a week to keep your hair hydrated and healthy. Different hair types will need different approaches. One way of developing a hair care routine is by following the tips that match your hair type and adjusting the routine where needed.

Tips for Straight Hair

Straight hair tends to be more oily and will need more frequent washing than other types of hair. Opt for a shampoo that will give your scalp a deep cleanse, and try to shampoo every two to three days. Sulfate-free shampoos are a good option. With conditioners, try to look for volumizing formulations to revitalize hair.

If you are using dry shampoo, select a product that will do double duty. For best results, go for dry shampoos that absorb oil and act as volumizers. Use the product in moderation, or it can weigh down your hair. Always apply a heat protector before using any heat tools.

Tips for Wavy Hair

This hair type needs to be washed less frequently, but it also requires a conditioner that hydrates the hair without weighing it down. It's advisable to avoid products that contain oils or heavy ingredients. Detangle your tresses in the shower and use deep conditioners as needed.

Use microfiber towels to minimize frizz when drying hair. To preserve the wavy texture, avoid combing or raking your hair when it's wet.

When applying products, start at the midpoint of your hair and use your palm to distribute them evenly. Air dry for effortless waves, or use a heat protection product if you need to use heat tools. A mousse can give waves extra definition and is preferable to gel.

Tips for Curly Hair

Dryness is a real danger for curly hair, so it is necessary to avoid using shampoos that exacerbate this problem. When choosing a conditioner, select products that will deeply moisturize your hair.

Deep conditioning at least once a week is essential to keeping curls in good condition.

To dry curly hair, use a microfiber towel to minimize frizz. Apply leave-in conditioner and style hair as desired. Gels and mousses can easily be scrunched into hair and provide lasting hold for curl definition.

Air dry your curls or speed things up with a hairdryer, but be sure to use a heat protectant if you do.

Tips for Coily Hair

Coily hair is easily damaged, so our hair care routine needs to lock moisture in the hair to prevent breakage. Be as gentle as possible with this hair type, and use sulfate-free shampoos.

Moisture-adding products high in humectants are a good option to add extra hydration to your hair. It's recommended to wash this hair type no more than twice a week. If you need to wash your hair more often, try co-washing between shampoo days.

Detangle your hair gently with your fingers when applying conditioner to minimize tangles. Use a deep conditioner at least once a week to keep your hair soft and shiny.

After washing and conditioning hair, consider using the LOC method (described in Chapter 4) to give hair an extra moisture boost.

Avoid using flat irons, hair dryers, and other hot tools as much as possible. It's best to let your hair air dry, but when that's not possible, use a diffuser attachment on your hair dryer. The hair dryer should be on the lowest heat setting. You may need to use a heat-protectant product before blow drying.

There is no one-size-fits-all solution to developing a hair care routine. Using products that are specifically designed for your hair type can make a huge difference in the health and appearance of your hair. For example, if you have curly hair, using a product designed for curly hair can help enhance your natural curls and reduce frizz.

Latina women have a wide range of hair types and textures, which means there are endless possibilities for styling and embracing your natural hair. Whether you have straight or curly hair, embrace the versatility of your hair and find what works best for you.

Experimenting With Different Hairstyles

Sometimes, we rock the same look for what feels like years. Other times, we may want to switch styles after a few weeks. Hairstyles come and go, but when we feel the need to change things up, it's best to pick a hairstylist that we are comfortable with. Experimenting with different hairstyles can help you find what works best for your hair type and face shape. Try out different braids, updos, and even hair accessories to find your perfect style. You can also consult a professional stylist for recommendations.

If you're not ready to commit to a new look but want to "try on" different styles, there's an app that can help. Several actually. These apps give us an idea of how different hairstyles and colors will look on us without having to undergo a big change just yet. Make a statement with your hairstyle! These tips will help you sport the freshest look on the block.

Add Playful Bangs

Just about any hairstyle can be transformed with bangs. From wispy and playful to bold and blocky, bangs are very versatile additions to a hairstyle. Some people try out bangs for a little while, while others wear them as a signature look. There's no denying that bangs lend a youthful, fun, and edgy look to a hairstyle. Sometimes, changing your bangs and the way you wear them is all that's needed to create a fresh and popping hairstyle. Bangs are stylish, but they are hard work and will need a regular trim to maintain their style and shape. Some ladies cut their own bangs. Learning this skill can be a great way to maintain bangs or to refresh a hairstyle we may have grown bored with. Here are some steps on how to cut bangs:

- **Wash your hair:** Start by washing your hair and letting it dry completely. This will help you to see how your hair naturally falls and avoid cutting it too short.

- **Choose the type of bangs you want:** There are several types of bangs, including straight, side-swept, and blunt. Choose the type of bangs that you like, and that will complement your face shape.

- **Section off your hair:** Use a comb to section off the hair you want to cut. Separate your bangs from the rest of your hair and clip the rest of your hair away.

- **Determine the length:** Use your fingers or a comb to determine the length of your bangs. Hold your hair to the point where you want to cut it and mark the length with your fingers or a hair clip.

- **Cut your bangs:** Use a pair of sharp scissors to cut your bangs. Start by making small cuts and work your way up to the desired length. Be careful not to cut your hair too short or unevenly.

- **Check your work:** After cutting your bangs, check your work in the mirror. Make any necessary adjustments to ensure that they are even and at the desired length.

- **Style your bangs:** Style your bangs using a blow dryer or a flat iron to achieve the desired look. You can also use styling products such as hairspray or mousse to help your bangs stay in place.

Remember, cutting your own bangs can be tricky, so if you are unsure or nervous, it's always best to go to a professional stylist.

Layers for Movement

Layers give flat hair movement and texture, but we need to consider our curls too. If a Latina with very curly hair wanted her hair cut in layers, she might end up with a round shape to her hair. Layers, when done right, can frame the face, give volume, and define the shape of our hair. They also make hair easier to manage and give a fuller appearance to thin hair.

Try a Statement Haircut

The bob is not going to fade out of fashion any time soon. This haircut can range from super chic to whimsically playful and suits most people beautifully. If you're considering a bob, get it cut to accent your face shape. For example, the weight line of the bob can draw attention to the jawline. Bob haircuts are a good choice when you feel you need to cut your hair but don't want to commit to anything that may be too short.

Go Old School

When it comes to textured, curly, and coily hair, one on-trend look is to embrace our hair in its natural state. A freehand cut by a seasoned hairstylist can create a lasting hairstyle for us to enjoy. It's a good idea to embrace your hair's natural state and give it a break from heat and chemical treatments.

Experiment With Accessories

A scrunchie or colorful clip can spice up a look in an instant. When selecting scrunchies, opt for silk or satin where possible. The idea is to minimize pulling on the hair as much as possible. Some hair ties have a tendency to rip out and damage our hair and should be avoided.

Want to bedazzle your do with a colorful clip? There are a few things to keep in mind when selecting hair accessories; after all, if a piece is both stylish and functional, it's a win in our books. Here are some things to look for:

- **Material:** Hair accessories can be made from a variety of materials, including plastic, metal, fabric, and wood. Choose a material that is comfortable to wear and fits the occasion.

- **Size:** Consider the size of the hair accessory in relation to your hair. Larger accessories can be more noticeable and add a statement to your look, while smaller ones can be more subtle and delicate.

- **Style:** Hair accessories come in a variety of styles, from classic to trendy. Consider your personal style and the occasion you will be wearing the accessory for when choosing the style.

- **Comfort:** Make sure the hair accessory is comfortable to wear and doesn't cause any discomfort or pain. Avoid accessories that are too tight or heavy.

- **Function:** Consider the function of the hair accessory. Will it hold your hair securely in place? Will it add volume or texture to your hair? Choose an accessory that meets your hair needs.

- **Color:** Choose a color that compliments your hair color and skin tone. A contrasting color can add a pop of color to your outfit, while a matching color can create a more cohesive look.

- **Durability:** Choose a hair accessory that is durable and can withstand daily wear and tear. Look for accessories that are well-made and have a sturdy construction.

By considering these factors, you can choose hair accessories that not only look great and spruce up a hairstyle but also function well and are comfortable to wear.

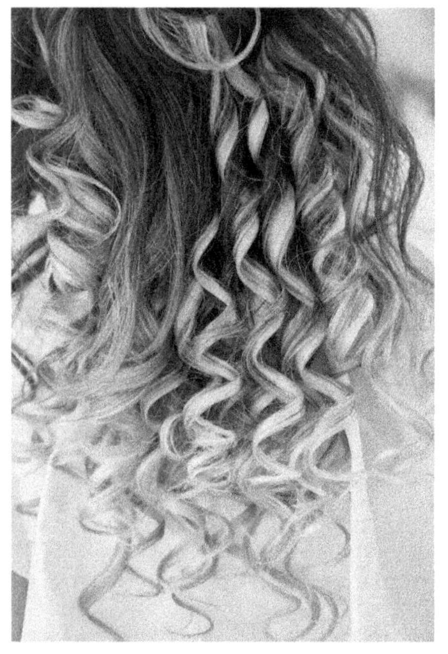

Amp Up Your Bun-Game

Buns are a staple, but that does not mean they have to be boring. If you've grown tired of a messy bun or don't quite feel the top knot, give this braided bun a try. The style works well on medium-length hair and longer.

Start with a ponytail. Make some braids with your hair. The amount and type of braid are up to you, but you'll need to fold the braids on top of each other and pin them in place to create the bun. Try experimenting with different braids when making the bun. Rope braids, fishtail braids, and Dutch braids give a different character to the hairstyle. Not only that, but different braids may hold differently in various hair types, so it is worth experimenting a bit to see what works best. A braided bun is a great hairstyle for most occasions, including weddings.

Try a Splash of Color

Nothing can refresh a hairstyle quite like a new color or some flattering highlights and lowlights. Subtle chocolate tones can enhance browns, making the color pop. That's because warm tones tend to reflect more light. However you wish to personalize your hair color, it is best to talk to a hairstylist before you do so. Tell the stylist which colors and tones you like and which ones you don't. Make sure your stylist understands what you mean by "copper," "auburn," or "burgundy," as they may have a different understanding of these and other colors.

As part of the search for a new style, experimenting with highlights can be a fun and effective way to freshen up your look. One way to do this is by applying lighter, softer dyes that don't require bleaching and don't contain harsh chemicals like amines, peroxides, or alcohol. These gentle dyes can help illuminate your face and give you a more youthful appearance.

When it comes to highlights, there are a variety of techniques and products to choose from. For example, you may want to consider small strands of non-permanent extensions, which can be a great way to add highlights without committing to a permanent change. These extensions can be easily removed when you're ready to change up your look again.

Whether you choose to use gentle dyes or non-permanent extensions, the key is to find a look that complements your natural features and enhances your overall appearance. Play around with different styles and colors until you find the perfect look for you. With a little experimentation and some expert guidance, you can achieve the highlights you've been dreaming of and enjoy a fresh new style that highlights your unique beauty.

Maintaining the Look

A new look will only stay fresh for so long before it needs maintenance. Maintenance can make the difference between loving your new do and desperately wishing for your hair to outgrow an undesirable hairstyle faster. If your hair is colored, you'll need color maintenance to keep the color vibrant. You may need specific products and tools to style the look as well, so we'll need to consider our budgets as well.

When we completely change our hairstyles, it can take some getting used to, especially when we've had the same style for a long time. Take your time to adjust to the new style and try not to revert to old habits that damage your hair. Above all, enjoy your new flattering look!

More Than Hair Care

Hair care can mean different things to different people. Some of us consider it a routine task, while others see it as an important part of our heritage and identity. While many people today opt for keratin treatments at salons, others follow their traditional hair care methods, which make them stand out. For instance, in India, coconut and almond oil are commonly used as a hair mask to moisturize naturally thick hair. This practice is rooted in Indian culture, which places high regard on hair as an essential aspect of beauty. Meanwhile, Danish women have a more relaxed approach to hair care, often opting for dry shampoos and hair masks, while Brazilian women splurge on keratin treatments to manage dry and frizzy hair (Hair by Moses, n.d.).

Each culture has unique hair care practices that make them stand out, and these practices continue to coexist alongside modern hair trends. So it would be helpful to surround yourself with positive influences that can help boost your confidence and self-esteem. This can include following social media accounts that promote natural hair, attending hair care events, or finding a supportive hair care community.

Hosting hair care parties with friends is a great way to bond and learn about new hair care techniques and products. You can invite friends over to share their own hair care routines and try out new products together. This is a fun and relaxed way to experiment with different hair care products and learn from each other's experiences. You can also make it a themed event, such as a natural hair care party or a DIY hair mask party.

Participating in online hair care communities is another great way to learn and share hair care tips and advice. Online communities can provide a supportive environment where you can connect with other Latina women who share similar hair types and learn from their experiences. You can ask questions, share your own tips, and get feedback on your hair care routine.

Attending hair care events and conferences is an excellent way to learn from professionals in the hair care industry. You can attend workshops and seminars to learn about new products and techniques for maintaining healthy and beautiful hair. You can also meet other Latina women who share similar hair types and learn new tips and tricks for managing your hair. Attending these events can be a great way to connect with others who are passionate about hair care and stay up-to-date on the latest trends and innovations in the industry.

Eleven

Conclusion

As Latinas, we have been conditioned to believe that natural hair is "*pelo malo*" and that it needs to be straightened, chemically treated, or hidden under wigs and weaves to be deemed acceptable. It's easy to fall into this mindset when the media and societal beauty standards perpetuate the idea. The lack of representation of diverse hair types in the beauty industry doesn't help either. However, it is time for us to take ownership of our beauty and embrace our natural hair, no matter the texture, length, or color. Your hair will thank you for it. Taking care of our hair involves:

- Regular washes

- Consistent conditioner use

- Avoiding heat

- Protecting hair from the sun

- Eating a balanced diet

- Going for regular trims

- Brushing your hair gently

- Avoiding damaging activities such as over-styling and over-washing hair

One way we can confidently embrace our natural hair is to arm ourselves with the knowledge and tools needed to care for it properly. This book aims to do just that by providing information on the different hair types and textures that Latina women may have, as well as tips and tricks for maintaining healthy, beautiful hair. By understanding the unique needs of our hair, we can learn how to care for it in a way that enhances its natural beauty rather than trying to alter it to fit into a narrow definition of beauty.

In addition to embracing our natural hair, it is important to promote diversity in the beauty industry as a whole. This means not only hiring more people of color in all aspects of the industry but also creating products that cater to a wider range of skin tones, hair types, and beauty needs. By doing so, beauty brands can ensure that everyone feels represented and included and that no one is left out or marginalized. As Latinas, we can also do our part to support and uplift each other as a community. This means celebrating each other's beauty, sharing tips and tricks for hair care, and advocating for more representation and inclusion in the beauty industry. We can also support small, independent beauty brands that are owned by Latinas and help promote and elevate their voices and products.

It is important to remember that we are stronger together than we are apart. By coming together as a community, we can create real change in the beauty industry and society as a whole. We can show the world that our natural hair is beautiful and worthy of celebration and that we are proud of who we are and where we come from.

Artemis Beauty

I feel proud to write for our Latino community.

— ♥ ♥ ♥ —

If you enjoyed reading my book, please leave me your review and recommend it. Your opinion is precious to me, as it motivates me to continue researching and developing knowledge that meets our specific needs.

Hughs.
Catalina

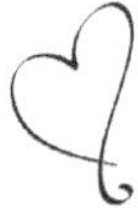

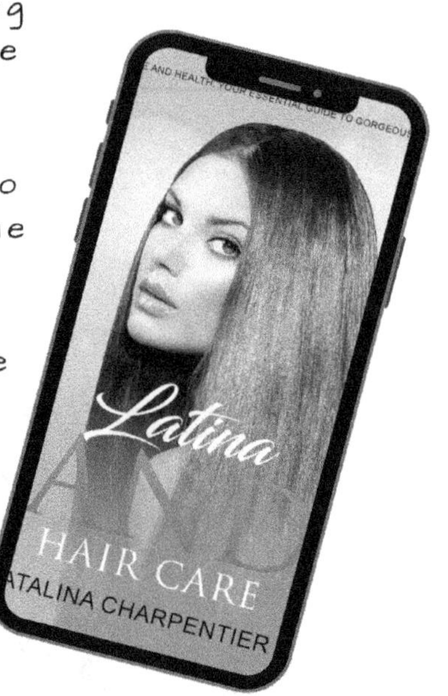

www.artemixbeauty.com

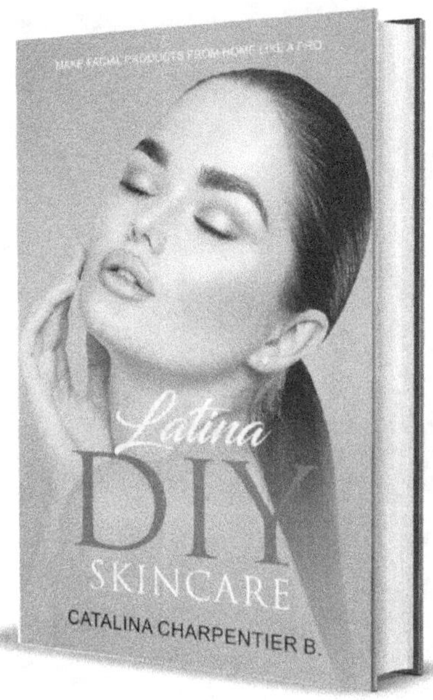

Take your Skincare to the next level! Discover how to create natural products like a professional from the comfort of your home.

www.artemixbeauty.com

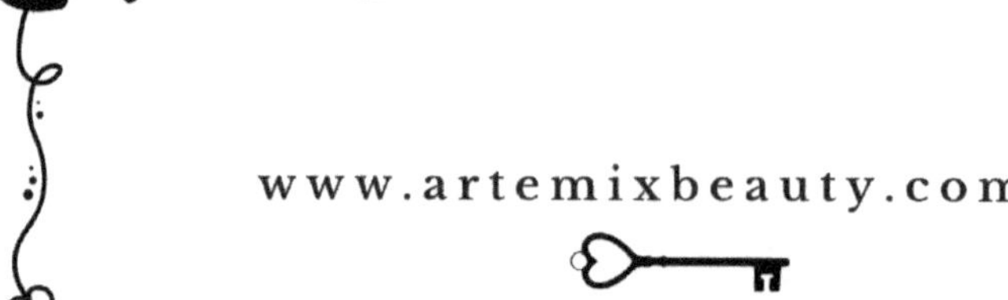

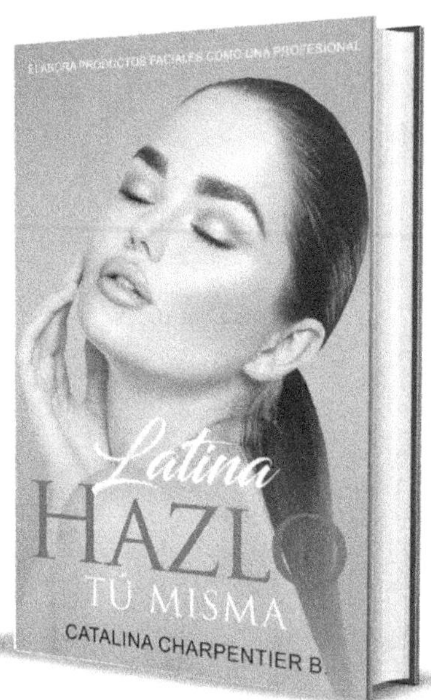

¡Lleva tu cuidado de la piel al siguiente nivel! Descubre cómo crear productos naturales como un profesional desde la comodidad de tu hogar.

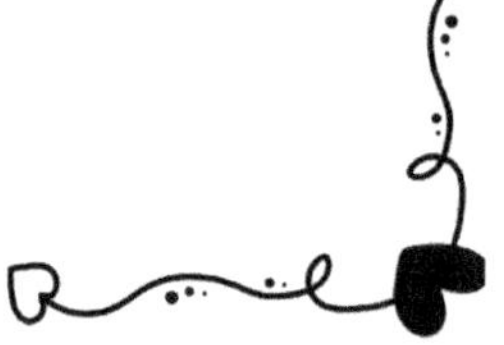

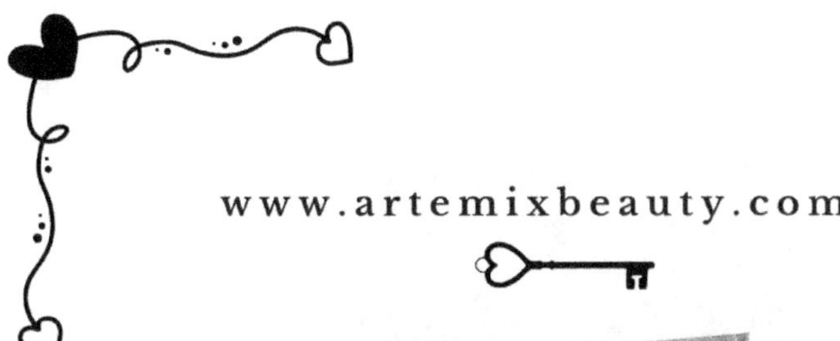

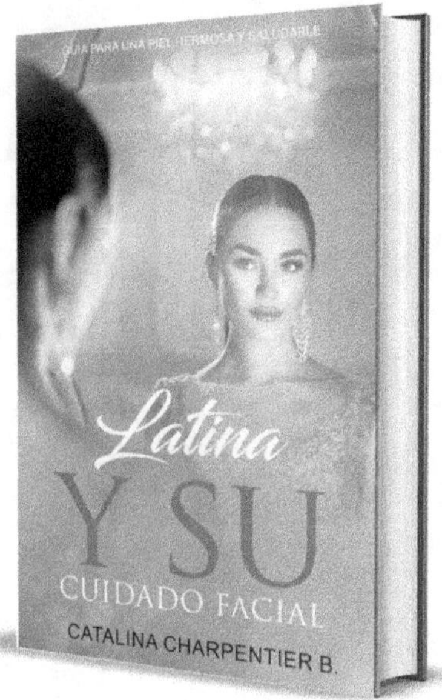

Descubre los secretos para lucir espectacular en cada página. Aprende sobre el cuidado de la piel, la elección de productos y los mejores suplementos para rejuvenecer tu rostro.

Twelve

References

Almohanna, H. M., Ahmed, A. A., Tsatalis, J. P., & Tosti, A. (2019). The role of vitamins and minerals in hair loss: A review. *Dermatology and Therapy, 9*(1), 51–70. https://doi.org/10.1 007/s13555-018-0278-6

American Academy of Dermatology. (n.d.-a). *Black hair: Tips for everyday care.* https://www.aad.org/public/everyday-care/hair-scal p-care/hair/care-african-american

American Academy of Dermatology. (n.d.-b). *Hairstyles that pull can lead to hair loss.* https://www.aad.org/public/diseases/hair-loss /causes/hairstyles

American Academy of Dermatology Association. (n.d.-c). *Do you have hair loss or hair shedding?* https://www.aad.org/public/diseas es/hair-loss/insider/shedding

Amra. (2016, April 22). *The dos and don'ts of deep conditioning: Make the most of your routine.* All Things

Hair. https://www.allthingshair.com/en-uk/hair-care/how-to-dee p-condition-hair/dos-donts-deep-conditioning/

Benefits of using hair masks: How does it help your hair? (2022, March 24). Innovist. https://innovist.com/blogs/all/benefits-of-using-hai r-masks

Better Health Channel. (n.d.). *Water—a vital nutrient.* Victoria State Government. https://www.betterhealth.vic.gov.au/health/he althyliving/water-a-vital-nutrient

BosleyMD. (n.d.). *How to keep your hair follicles healthy.* https://bosleymd.com/blogs/hair-thinning/how-to-keep -your-hair-follicles-healthy

Bradshaw, H. (2022, December 4). *Rosemary is the secret to long and healthy hair. Here's how to use it to grow luscious locks.* Popular Science. https://www.popsci.com/diy/rosemary-water-for-hair/#:~ :text=Green%20explains%20that%20rosemary%20owes

Brady, K. (2019, November 18). *11 ways to use jojoba oil for healthier skin and hair, according to dermatologists.* Prevention. https://ww w.prevention.com/beauty/a29829814/jojoba-oil-benefits/

Can the amount of water you drink affect hair loss and growth? (n.d.). MedicineNet. https://www.medicinenet.com/amount_of_water_ drink_affect_hair_loss_and_growth/article.htm

Capric triglyceride in hair care products. (n.d.). Anveya. https://www.anveya.com/blogs/top-tips/capric-triglyceride-in-hair-care-products

Castañon, K. (2017, October 11). *It's time we talked about the term "pelo malo."* Refinery29. https://www.refinery29.com/en-us/2017/10/166300/latin-american-hair-pelo-malo-meaning-history

Catcher, J. (2021, April 7). *This $10 hair oil can help you regrow strands in just 8 days.* Woman's World. https://www.womansworld.com/posts/beauty/spanish-almond-oil-for-hair-growth

Cherney, K. (2023, February 14). *How to stop hair breakage.* Healthline. https://www.healthline.com/health/hair-breakage

Collins-Hermanstein, C. (n.d.). *The benefits of using honey on natural hair.* Curls Understood. https://curlsunderstood.com/benefits-of-honey-for-natural-hair/

Cook, H. (2019, January 7). *10 reasons to choose natural hair products this year.* Bouclème. https://www.boucleme.co.uk/blogs/news/natural-hair-products-benefits

Darbre, P. D., Aljarrah, A., Miller, W. R., Coldham, N. G., Sauer, M. J., & Pope, G. S. (2004). Concentrations of parabens in human breast tumours. *Journal of Applied Toxicology: JAT, 24*(1), 5–13. https://doi.org/10.1002/jat.958

Davidson, K. (2021, May 3). *Hair vitamins: What are they, and do they work?* Healthline. https://www.healthline.com/nutrition/do-hair-vitamins-work#bottom-line

De Bellefonds, C. (2021, April 14). *Goodbye, dry hair: Here's how to deep condition at home like a pro.* Healthline. https://www.healthline.com/health/beauty-skin-care/how-to-deep-condition-hair

Derreck, J. (2021, April 23). *Your face shape can help you find your perfect hairstyle—here's how.* Byrdie. https://www.byrdie.com/why-face-shape-matters-when-choosing-a-hairstyle-346355

Derreck, J. (2022, May 25). *How to choose the perfect haircut for face shape.* Byrdie. https://www.byrdie.com/how-to-choose-the-perfect-haircut-for-your-hair-texture-and-face-shape-346346

Dixon, M. (2013, July 22). *Myth or fact: Coconut oil is an effective sunscreen.* Mayo Clinic Health System. https://mayoclinichealthsystem.org/hometown-health/speaking-of-health/myth-or-fact-coconut-is-an-effective-sunscreen

Dry Scalp vs. Dandruff. (n.d.). L'Oreal Professionnel. https://www.lorealprofessionnel.co.uk/hair-advice/hair-care-advice/dry-scalp-vs-dandruff#:~:text=While%20dry%20skin%20accompanies%20dry

Felton, K. (2020, January 9). *The best hair straightening brushes that will make you break up with your flat iron.* Shape.

https://www.shape.com/lifestyle/beauty-style/best-hair-straighteni
ng-brushes#:~:text=Straightening%20brushes%20tend%20to%20be

Folate (folic ccid)—vitamin B9. (n.d.). Harvard School of Public
Health. https://www.hsph.harvard.edu/nutritionsource/folic-acid/

Frothingham, S. (2019, September 27). *Benefits of fish oil for hair and
how to use.* Healthline. https://www.healthline.com/health/fish-oil
-for-hair

Gardener, S. S. (2021, November 15). *Facts about gray hair.* Web-
MD. https://www.webmd.com/beauty/ss/slideshow-beauty-gray
-hair-facts#:~:text=Your%20hair%20follicles%20have%20pigment

Gavazzoni Dias, M. F. (2015). Hair cosmetics: An overview. *International Journal of Trichology, 7*(1), 2–15. https://doi.org/10.4103/0
974-7753.153450

Gómez, S. (2017, October 10). *Hispanic HAIR-itage: Find best
products to use according to your texture, plus quick how-tos.* Latin
Times. https://www.latintimes.com/hispanic-hair-itage-find-best
-products-use-according-your-texture-plus-quick-how-tos-425369

Gonzalez, I. (2014, December 24). *10 things only Latina girls understand about beauty.* SheKnows. https://www.sheknows.com/living
/articles/1067357/latina-girls-know-beauty/

Gould, H. (2022, August 26). *Peppermint oil for hair: Benefits and
how to use it.* Byrdie. https://www.byrdie.com/peppermint-oil-for
-hair#:~:text=%22Peppermint%20oil%20helps%20to%20stimulate

Guerra, J. (2022, March 4). *The 12 best hair brushes for curly hair, according to experts.* WWD. https://wwd.com/shop/shop-beauty/best-curly-hair-brushes-1235093848/

Gupta, A. (2019, December 5). *Dull skin, falling hair? A folic acid deficiency might be the cause.* Vogue India. https://www.vogue.in/wellness/content/benefits-of-folic-acid-for-hair-loss-glowing-skin-vitamin-b9-hair-growth-supplements

Gupta, S. (2020, September 16). *Green tea is the "secret" remedy for hair loss. Here's how you can use it.* Healthshots. https://www.healthshots.com/beauty/hair-care/green-tea-is-the-secret-remedy-for-hair-loss-heres-how-you-can-use-it/

Hair by Moses. (n.d.). *Hair care around the world: How different cultures take care of their hair.* https://www.hairbymoses.com/blog/hair-care-around-the-world-how-different-cultures-take-care-of-their-hair/

Hair science p2: The hair types. (2023, March 2). Essentially Natural. https://essentiallynatural.co.za/blogs/the-essentially-natural-blog/hair-science-p2-the-hair-types

Hannah. (2018, June 13). *How to use argan oil + DIY serum recipe for vibrant hair.* Mountainrose Herbs. https://blog.mountainroseherbs.com/how-to-use-argan-oil

Heat-damaged hair; how heat can affect the health of your hair. (n.d.). Hair Flair. https://www.hairflair.com/2022/05/06/heat-damaged -hair/

Hill, M. (n.d.). *DIY dry shampoo for any hair colour.* Mums at the Table. https://mumsatthetable.com/diy-dry-shampoo/

Hjalmarsdottir, F. (2023, January 17). *17 science-based benefits of omega-3 fatty acids.* Healthline. https://www.healthline.com/nutr ition/17-health-benefits-of-omega-3#TOC_TITLE_HDR_8

Honey for hair: The benefits and how to use it. (n.d.) . Gisou. https://gisou.com/blogs/blog/honey-for-hair#:~:text=It% 20turns%20out%20that%20honey

How does heat damage hair? (n.d.). Dyson. https://www.dyson.com/knowledge/hair-care/how-does-heat-dam age-hair#:~:text=Exposure%20to%20high%20heat%20changes

How to properly apply your hair product. (2019, August 16). TouchUps Salon. https://www.touchupssalon.com/how-to-prope rly-apply-your-hair-product/

How to use shea butter for hair and skin. (n.d.). Garnier. https://www.garnierusa.com/tips-how-tos/how-shea-butter-impro ves-your-skin-and-hair#:~:text=Use%20a%20small%20amount%20 of

How to use the LOC method. (n.d.). LUSH. https://www.lushusa.c om/stories/article-how-to-use-the-LOC-method.html

Importance of choosing the right shampoo for your hair type. (n.d.). UltraSoft. https://www.theultrasoft.in/importance-of-choosing-the-right-shampoo-for-your-hair-type/

John, N. (2022, May 31). *15 unique Latina hairstyles that are always in trend.* HairstylesFeed. https://hairstylesfeed.com/latina-hairstyles/

Julson, E. (2023, April 4). *15 signs and symptoms of vitamin C deficiency.* Healthline. https://www.healthline.com/nutrition/vitamin-c-deficiency-symptoms#TOC_TITLE_HDR_15

Khalfe, F. (2022, August 2). *More than just a mane: Exploring the cultural symbolism of hair in womanhood.* Glamour. https://www.glamour.co.za/beauty/hair/more-than-just-a-mane-exploring-the-cultural-symbolism-of-hair-in-womanhood-a1e73b50-02af-4972-a08b-847ebeb404b4

Kilikita, J. (2022, September 28). *The looped bun: A TikTok tutorial for every hair type.* Refinery29. https://www.refinery29.com/en-us/looped-bun-hairstyle-tutorial

Kunin, A. (n.d.). *How to protect your hair from the elements.* DERMAdoctor. https://www.dermadoctor.com/blog/how-to-protect-your-hair-from-the-elements/

La Jeunesse, M. (2020, May 15). *9 Latina women with great hair share their secrets.* Glamour. https://www.glamour.com/story/latina-hair-care-tips

Le Floc'h, C., Cheniti, A., Connétable, S., Piccardi, N., Vincenzi, C., & Tosti, A. (2015). Effect of a nutritional supplement on hair loss in women. *Journal of Cosmetic Dermatology, 14*(1), 76–82. https://doi.org/10.1111/jocd.12127

Manso, J. (2021, April 16). *Black, Hispanic shoppers driving beauty sales, according to NielsenIQ.* WWD. https://wwd.com/feature/black-hispanic-shoppers-driving-beauty-sales-according-to-nielseniq-1234800340/

Marczuk, J. (n.d.). *10 toxic ingredients to avoid in your hair products.* Love Hair. https://lovehair.com/blogs/the-daily-muse/harmful-ingredients

MedlinePlus. (n.d.). *Vitamin C.* https://medlineplus.gov/ency/article/002404.htm

Moor, O. (2022, September 14). *30 sexy Latina hairstyles we love in 2023.* You Probably Need a Haircut. https://youprobablyneedahaircut.com/latina-hairstyles/

Myths and tips about protective styles! (2021, June 10). NaturAll. https://naturallclub.com/blogs/the-naturall-club-blog/myths-and-tips-about-protective-styles

Nall, R. (2018, May 22). *How to use essential oils for hair growth.* Medical News Today. https://www.medicalnewstoday.com/articles/32187

Oh, J. Y., Park, M. A., & Kim, Y. C. (2014). Peppermint oil promotes hair growth without toxic signs. *Toxicological Research, 30*(4), 297–304. https://doi.org/10.5487/tr.2014.30.4.297

Pai, D. (2016, March 3). *9 sneaky hair-washing mistakes you're making*. Glamour. https://www.glamour.com/story/common-mistakes-washing-hair-shampoo-conditioner

Palomares, S. (2015, March 3). *20 Latina celeb haircuts that never go out of style*. Mamas Latinas. https://mamaslatinas.com/beauty-style/134107-20_latina_celeb_haircuts_that

Panahi, Y., Taghizadeh, M., Marzony, E. T., & Sahebkar, A. (2015). Rosemary oil vs minoxidil 2% for the treatment of androgenetic alopecia: a randomized comparative trial. *Skinmed, 13*(1), 15–21. https://pubmed.ncbi.nlm.nih.gov/25842469/

Panthenol (pro-vitamin B5). (n.d.). CurlyEllie. https://www.curlyellie.com/pages/panthenol-pro-vitamin-b5#:~:text=Pro%20Vitamin%20B5%20or%20D

Patel, D. P., Swink, S. M., & Castelo-Soccio, L. (2017). A review of the use of biotin for hair loss. *Skin Appendage Disorders, 3*(3), 166–169. https://doi.org/10.1159/000462981

Petre, A. (2019, November 28). *6 benefits and uses of omega-3s for skin and hair*. Healthline. Healthline. https://www.healthline.com/nutrition/omega-3-benefits-on-skin-and-hair

Pitman, S. (2018, August 16). *What's happening in the Latin America hair care market? Part I.* CosmeticsDesign. https://www.cosmeticsdesign.com/Article/2018/08/15/What-s-happening-in-the-Latin-America-hair-care-market-Part-I

Raman, R. (2022, May 18). *The 13 best foods for hair growth.* Healthline. https://www.healthline.com/nutrition/foods-for-hair-growth

Raypole, C. (2019, August 27). *4 nourishing DIY olive oil hair masks.* Healthline. https://www.healthline.com/health/olive-oil-hair-mask

Roeschley, A. A. (2015, July 9). *What's influencing Latinas in the beauty aisle?* Global Cosmetic Industry. https://www.gcimagazine.com/consumers-markets/article/21850044/whats-influencing-latinas-in-the-beauty-aisle

Russick, J. (n.d.). *Hair cuticle: Understanding this important part of your hair.* Function of Beauty. https://www.functionofbeauty.com/blog/lightreads/hair-cuticle/

Santos-Longhurst, A. (2019, February 22). *Does argan oil help protect against hair loss?* Healthline. https://www.healthline.com/health/argan-oil-for-hair-growth#overview

SciTechDaily. (2022, July 9). *6 vitamins to transform your dry, damaged hair into perfect glossy locks.* https://scitechdaily.com/6-vitamins-to-transform-your-dry-damaged-hair-into-perfect-glossy-locks/#:~:text=Vitamin%20A%20also%20helps%20your

7 signs of heat-damaged hair & 3 ways to revive it. (2023, January 20). NuMe. https://numehair.com/es/blogs/hair-care/signs-of-heat-damaged-hair

Smith, J. (2018, January 18). *Traction alopecia: Symptoms and prevention.* Medical News Today. https://www.medicalnewstoday.com/articles/320648

Smith, S. L., Choueiti, M., Pieper, K., Case, A., Yao, K., & Choi, A. (2017). *Inequality in 900 popular films: Examining portrayals of gender, race, ethnicity, LGBTQ, and disability from 2007–2016.* USC Annenberg https://annenberg.usc.edu/sites/default/files/Dr_Stacy_L_Smith-Inequality_in_900_Popular_Films.pdf

Soni, A. (2022, September 9). *Is glycerin good for your hair?* Vedix. https://vedix.com/blogs/articles/how-to-use-glycerin-on-your-hair#:~:text=Glycerin%20is%20one%20of%20the%20best%20natural%20conditioners%20for%20the

Stanborough, R. J. (2019-a, August 28). *Can using dry shampoo damage your hair?* Healthline. https://www.healthline.com/health/is-dry-shampoo-bad-for-your-hair

Stanborough, R. J. (2019-b, August 30). *How to identify and style your hair type.* Healthline. https://www.healthline.com/health/beauty-skin-care/types-of-hair#the-takeaway

The ancient powers and benefits of olive oil for hair. (n.d.). Garnier. https://www.garnier.ca/en-ca/tips-and-how-tos/the-ancient-powers-and-benefits-of-olive-oil-for-hair

The Healthy Journal. (n.d.). *Frequently asked questions*. https://www.thehealthyjournal.com/q-and-a/how-often-should-you-trim-your-hair-to-avoid-split-ends#:~:text=Unless%20you%20are%20growing%20your

Trüeb, R. (2016). Serum biotin levels in women complaining of hair loss. *International Journal of Trichology, 8*(2), 73. https://doi.org/10.4103/0974-7753.188040

UV and Your Hair. (2022, February 2). Colleen. https://www.colleen.nz/archive/uv-and-your-hair#:~:text=Hair%20lipids%20are%20damaged%20by

Watson, K. (2019, March 8). *What is shea butter? 22 reasons to add it to your routine*. Healthline. https://www.healthline.com/health/beauty-skin-care/what-is-shea-butter#dandruff

Watson, K. (2023, April 20). *Aloe vera for your hair: What are the benefits?* Healthline. https://www.healthline.com/health/aloe-vera-for-hair#:~:text=Strengthens%20and%20repairs%20hair%20strands

Weimert, K. (2020, August 21). *How often should you condition your hair?* Healthline. https://www.healthline.com/health/how-often-should-you-condition-your-hair#takeaway

West, H. (2021, August 25). *Coconut oil for your hair: Benefits, uses and tips*. Healthline. https://www.healthline.com/nutrition/cocon ut-oil-and-hair

What is hair mousse & how to use it. (n.d.). Nexxus. https://www.n exxus.com/us/en/haircare-101/what-is-hair-mousse/

What is hair pH and why is it important for your hair. (2022, May 10). Redken. https://www.redken.com/blog/haircare/why-the-ph-of-your-hair-i s-important#:~:text=So%2C%20What%20Happens%20if%20Hair

White, A. (2017, September 29). *Jojoba oil for hair: How it works*. Healthline. https://www.healthline.com/health/jojoba-oil-for-hair #considerations

White, A. (2018, November 14). Can peppermint oil benefit your hair? Healthline. https://www.healthline.com/health/peppermint -oil-for-hair#benefits

White, A. (2022, September 15). *Should I use rosemary oil for hair growth?* Healthline. https://www.healthline.com/health/rosemary -oil-for-hair

White, A. (2023, March 13). *Can apple cider vinegar benefit your hair?* Healthline. https://www.healthline.com/health/apple-cider -vinegar-hair#benefits

Wong, C. (2022, August 31). *What you need to know about using coconut oil for your hair*. Verywell Health. https://www.verywellhealth.com/coconut-oil-for-your-hair-4171883

Woodford, B. (2020, July 8). *How to protect your natural hair from sun damage*. NaturallyCurly. https://www.naturallycurly.com/curlreading/curls/how-to-protect-your-natural-hair-from-sun-damage

Wright, J. (2022, February 4). *Black Latinas who broke barriers by embracing their natural hair*. Ceremonia. https://ceremonia.com/blogs/all/black-latinas-who-broke-barriers-by-embracing-their-natural-hair

Yang, F.-C., Zhang, Y., & Rheinstädter, M. C. (2014). The structure of people's hair. *PeerJ, 2*, e619. https://doi.org/10.7717/peerj.619

Image References

Alexander Krivitskiy. (2018, September, 10). *Grayscale of woman*. Pexels. https://www.pexels.com/photo/grayscale-of-woman-1406722/

Chef Akey. (2021, June, 29). *Vegetable salad on brown paper bowl*. Pexels. https://www.pexels.com/photo/vegetable-salad-on-brown-paper-bowl-8535717/

Cottonbro Studio. (2020, March, 23). *Black and gray corded devices*. Pexels. https://www.pexels.com/photo/black-and-gray-corded-devices-3992848/

Cottonbro Studio. (2020, March, 23). *Silver and black keys on brown wooden table*. Pexels. https://www.pexels.com/photo/silver-and-black-keys-on-brown-wooden-table-3993294/

Cottonbro Studio. (2021, April, 07). *A conditioner bottle near a hairpin*. Pexels. https://www.pexels.com/photo/a-conditioner-bottle-near-a-hairpin-7428103/

Cottonbro Studio. (2021, April, 08). *Photo of a conditioner container with barettes*. Pexels. https://www.pexels.com/photo/photo-of-a-conditioner-container-with-barettes-7440059/

Engin Akyurt. (2019, October, 11). *Photo of hairstyle*. Pexels. https://www.pexels.com/photo/photo-of-hairstyle-3065207/

Karolina Grabowska. (2020, March, 31). *Set of pink petals and bottle on table*. Pexels. https://www.pexels.com/photo/set-of-pink-petals-and-bottle-on-table-4041231/

Karolina Grabowska. (2020, August, 31). *Woman washing her hair*. Pexels. https://www.pexels.com/photo/woman-washing-her-hair-5241036/

La Miko. (2020, February, 04). *Woman in black hat sitting in front of glass window*. Pexels. https://www.pexels.com/photo/woman-in-black-hat-sitting-in-front-of-glass-window-3681653/

Mareefe. (2018, November, 27). *Clear glass bowl beside yellow flower*. Pexels. https://www.pexels.com/photo/clear-glass-bowl-beside-yellow-flower-1638280/

Nappy. (2019, January, 08). *Woman sitting on stair.* Pexels. https://www.pexels.com/photo/woman-sitting-on-stair-1771383/

Nataliya Vaitkevich. (2021, June, 24). *Hair products laying on a hair.* Pexels https://www.pexels.com/photo/hair-products-laying-on-a-hair-8467970/

Pavel Danilyuk. (2021, March, 18). *A woman in white long sleeve shirt holding a blue camera.* Pexels. https://www.pexels.com/photo/a-woman-in-white-long-sleeve-shirt-holding-a-blue-camera-7180886/

Pera Detlic. (2017, May, 19). *Woman wearing hat in grayscale photography.* Pixabay. https://pixabay.com/photos/fashion-woman-hat-portrait-2309519/

Pexels LATAM. (2023, March, 29). *An attractive woman kissing a vintage camera.* Pexels. https://www.pexels.com/photo/an-attractive-woman-kissing-a-vintage-camera-16135587/

Pixabay. (2016, October, 23) *Spilled bottle of yellow capsule pills.* Pexels. https://www.pexels.com/photo/spilled-bottle-of-yellow-capsule-pills-208518/

Polina Tankilevitch. (2020, February, 14). *Plastic bottles on shelf.* Pexels. https://www.pexels.com/photo/plastic-bottles-on-shelf-3735657/

RDNE Productions. (2022, June, 06). *Woman holding a hairdryer.* Pexels. https://www.pexels.com/photo/woman-holding-a-hairdryer-12405527/

Shopify Partners. (n.d.). *A stylist measures before cutting photo.* Burst. https://burst.shopify.com/photos/a-stylist-measures-before-cutting?q=hair+spray